"You don't have to be a mother or even a woman to be fascinated by the science and physiology that Garbes writes about." —Terry Gross, NPR's *Fresh Air*

"In spite of how long women have been giving birth, there is a lot of misinformation out there about pregnancy and motherhood. Angela Garbes seeks to get it straight in *Like a Mother*. She not only corrects misinformation but also offers advice and support." —*Bustle*

"The science is sublime. I especially appreciated, oddly, learning how much we still don't know about the high-stakes path to parenthood. But what got me was Garbes's regard for mothers as people in their own right, rather than the hosts or self-sacrificing caregivers they're conditioned to be." —*Seattle Times*

"*Like a Mother* is a deeply researched history of human reproduction; it is a jewel-bright memoir; it is hard science beautifully translated; it is funny; it is intersectional; it will crack you open and fill you with awe. Required reading for mothers, and doubly required for everyone else." —Lindy West, author of *Shrill*

D1167269

"Garbes examines preconceived ideas about pregnancy and the history of women's health from a critical standpoint, revealing the prejudices and politics so ingrained in our culture that they still affect the care (or lack thereof) pregnant women receive today. *Like a Mother* is a compelling read."

—*The Stranger* (Seattle)

"Garbes unpacks reams of pregnancy advice, often absurd in its conflicting demands. *Like a Mother* gave me a toolkit for approaching a hoped-for future." —*Huffington Post*

"The pregnancy book that every smart, feminist woman has been waiting for has finally arrived! Garbes's natural curiosity and enthusiasm is infectious and never sacrificed as she navigates the culture of pregnancy and once-taboo subjects like miscarriage, placentas, and the pelvic floor with humor and delight. Garbes insists, rightly and beautifully, that women deserve more: more information, more compassion, more autonomy as well as more support. I read *Like a Mother* in one sitting, and read half of it out loud to my husband. I finished the book filled with hope and gratitude, convinced this book is both necessary and long overdue."

—Meaghan O'Connell, author of *And Now We Have Everything*

"*Like a Mother* gives women straight talk on pregnancy, their bodies, and life after giving birth." —GMA.com

"An empowering resource. . . . Garbes shares up-to-date, well-substantiated information about women's physical and mental health, aiming to help readers reduce their anxiety and make truly informed choices."

—*Publishers Weekly*

"*Like a Mother* is the evidence-based, open-minded book that US pregnancy culture needs. . . . A true feminist accomplishment that puts trust and agency back with women and parents."

—*Rewire.News*

"Personal yet wildly informative, Garbes's book is about all the things you didn't know about pregnancy. Along the way, I realized just how little we know about the process of carrying a child until it happens to us, if it does."

—*Washington Post's* "The Lily"

"An instantly seminal book. . . . *Like a Mother* showcases Garbes's intellectual curiosity as much as it does her empathy."

—*Health*

"Angela Garbes's book will change how we talk about childbirth."

—*Pacific Standard*

"[*Like a Mother*] is many things: memoir, popular science, journalism. It is also a deeply political book that seamlessly blends anecdotes about topics like postpartum sex with a robust defense of reproductive rights and critiques of American health care policy."

—*Public Books*

LIKE A MOTHER

A FEMINIST JOURNEY
THROUGH THE SCIENCE AND CULTURE
OF PREGNANCY

ANGELA GARBES

HARPER WAVE
An Imprint of HarperCollins*Publishers*

FIRST HARPER WAVE PAPERBACK EDITION PUBLISHED 2019.

Library of Congress Cataloging-in-Publication Data has been applied for.

ISBN 978-0-06-266295-8 (pbk.)

22 23 LSC 10

For Mom and Noli Jo, who made me

"Nothing is more tenacious than the life we are made of."

—OCTAVIA BUTLER

CONTENTS

PART III: A NEW YOU

INTRODUCTION

The moment I found out I was pregnant, I was hungover. While epic evenings of drinking were mostly behind me (after I hit thirty, my hangovers had morphed into cruel, multiday affairs), the previous night had been a rare, fun exception. I was sleeping it off, my heavy breathing interrupted by the ring of my cell phone.

The night before, my husband and I had martinis at our house before heading to our favorite neighborhood restaurant for a pizza with anchovies and pickled peppers. I'd lost a pregnancy a couple of months prior, and a big part of our grieving process had been to give ourselves a break from focusing on anything baby-related. So, embracing our ability to act spontaneously, we ended up having a big night out like the ones we used to have when we were first getting to know each other and falling in love. Conversation, laughter, and affection (also cocktails and wine) flowed in the familiar, easy way that they had not in the weeks following my miscarriage. After dinner, we decided not to go home. We went to a '90s

R & B night at a club; I drank tequila and danced to Mariah Carey.

When my doctor called with the news the next morning, it felt as though my barely conscious brain had been jolted awake. During the months after my miscarriage, my period had not returned (and, let's be honest, we weren't having much sex anyway), so the possibility of pregnancy wasn't on my radar. When I saw the number on my phone screen, I scrambled out of bed and tried to pull myself together, as though he might actually be able to see me over the phone. I was in no condition for this.

"Hello!" I said with forced energy. The fake sound of my own voice startled me. "Hello, hi, this is Angela," I tried again.

"Good morning, Angela."

As soon as I heard his voice—unnervingly calm—I stopped moving. I'd recently had blood drawn to measure the level of the pregnancy hormone hCG (human chorionic gonadotropin) in my body. The test was supposed to offer insight as to whether my uterus was back to its pre-pregnancy state or if it was still holding on to any "retained products of conception," the clinical term for the placental and fetal tissue that can remain after a miscarriage. If the test results revealed the latter, I might need a surgical procedure of dilation and curettage (D and C) to "completely evacuate" my uterus. What I was hoping to hear was that my hCG level was back to zero, that my uterus was empty. That my cycle—and my life—could finally go back to normal.

My doctor cleared his throat. "I think you're pregnant," he said.

"No, I don't think so," I replied confidently, dismissively. He paused.

"Sorry, let me start over. Angela, this is your doctor calling. I'm calling to tell you that you are pregnant. Last week, your hCG level was six. Today it is 1,033. The only way that happens is pregnancy."

It was as though he had whispered an electric secret in my ear. The unexpected news was a pulsing live wire that I could neither control nor ignore. Pregnancy's current raced through me, giving off sparks of uncertainty and possibility. My mind flooded with an endless stream of questions, including a panicked, "Did I just pickle my embryo with tequila?"

Immediately after hanging up the phone, I began Googling.

"You may have heard that an occasional alcoholic drink is okay, but it's best to be on the safe side when you've got a baby on board," I read on the *What to Expect When You're Expecting* website.[1] "Why? Alcohol enters your baby's bloodstream in the same concentration as yours—and takes twice as long to leave it—so whatever you're drinking, your baby's downing one, too."

Uh-oh.

"But what about that night out with the girls (and a few too many margaritas) a couple of days before you found out you were pregnant?" the next sentence continued. "It happens to many moms, and (what a relief!) there's no need to worry."

Whew. Wait, what?

The rules on my computer screen seemed definitive yet contradictory, vaguely rooted in science yet pulled from the ether. I consider myself a generally calm and sensible person, but just minutes into this pregnancy, I was reeling with paranoia and confusion. I worried that the alcohol I had consumed the night before had already damaged the fragile (sesame seed–size, according to BabyCenter) life-form inside me, one I had spent the last months wondering if my thirty-six-year-old, past-its-reproductive-prime body and dusty, cobweb-lined uterus could even support.

This was my first clue that over the next two years, I would have many more questions than there would be sufficient answers.

My hunger for information was insatiable. I turned to books—classics like *What to Expect When You're Expecting* and the Sears *The Healthy Pregnancy Book* and *The Baby Book*—as well as online communities such as BabyCenter, The Bump, and What to Expect. I was looking for guidance, but after hours of reading through posts that used a strange lexicon of acronyms I didn't recognize (BBT, EBM, IC, LO, TTC) and texts that felt outdated, I never felt like I was being spoken to—and I still didn't have answers to my questions. These resources are written by doctors and mothers who present their opinions as definitive, which, as someone whose experiences fell outside those lines, left me feeling insecure, overwhelmed, and, often, judged.

If you've ever leafed through the pages of a pregnancy guidebook, you know what I'm talking about—the subtle (and not so subtle) finger-wagging implicit in even the most innocuous-seeming advice:

Scientific research has not yet determined whether cell phone radiation is harmful to mother or baby. Don't wait for the science to be "conclusive." Certainly don't sit around with your tablet or your cell phone propped up on your belly. Even stashing your cell phone in your purse may be too close.

Don't put any plastic containers in the microwave; choose glass or ceramic instead. Think about what is important to you and how you want to honor this very special time in your life. Be a strong "mama bear" and focus on protecting yourself and your baby.[2]

This attitude isn't limited to books—just look at the way pregnancy and motherhood are typically portrayed in popular movies and television shows. In American culture, motherhood is inextricably tied to the language of morality. Over and over, the message reinforced to expecting mothers is that there's a "right" and a "wrong" way to do things: You are a supposedly "good mom" if you abstain from caffeine and alcohol while pregnant, don't gain excess weight, plan a so-called natural childbirth (for the record, I believe that all birth is natural, no matter how it happens), breast-feed for at least a year, and glow with happiness throughout the whole process. You are a "bad mom" if you have the occasional glass of wine during pregnancy, experience anxiety or ambivalence about having a baby, look forward to an epidural, feed your baby formula, or take a pull off a joint once the kids are in bed because children are exhausting. This cultural standard is so well established that we even joke about it, proudly proclaiming ourselves "bad moms" when we stray from these expectations. We are trying to reclaim a term that we'd be much better off abandoning.

During pregnancy and the first few months of my daughter's life, by far the best advice I received came not from books or websites but from other pregnant women and new mothers. Some of them were close friends (or their older sisters) who lived across the country, others were friends of friends, people I barely knew. In pregnancy and motherhood we found camaraderie, a feeling that we were in the trenches together. We didn't necessarily have hard science to explain such perplexing phenomena as getting a transverse or breech fetus to turn head down, cluster feeding, perpetually leaky and/or saggy breasts and vaginas, and the slow healing of C-section incisions, but we had our own experiences and instincts. We were an army fighting for sanity and information. We texted back and forth at all hours of the day and night.

These frantic texts led me to deeper questions about female physiology and biology, as well as our society's expectations of and policies toward mothers. Questions about breast-feeding, in particular, nagged at me. I'd been told over and over that breast-feeding was best for babies, especially if they were sick, because breast milk was "good for immunity." But no health-care provider or book ever articulated exactly how or why breast milk helped babies' immune systems.

I wanted to breast-feed and, luckily, it went pretty smoothly for me and my daughter. But I had friends whose bodies were less cooperative, whose work environments were not accommodating of pumping milk, or who simply enjoyed the convenience of formula feeding. Their babies, like mine, were happy, healthy, and thriving. Considering that during the first few months of my daughter's life I spent more than eight hours a day, both at home and at work, breast-feeding and pumping, my body exhausted, sore, and depleted, I felt I was owed a better explanation.

But the answers to my questions couldn't be found at the doctor's office, either. That's because so much about female bodies—though they play the most crucial role in the continuation of our species—remains mysterious. We still haven't even managed to figure out what exactly starts labor—the physical process by which every single human is brought into the world. The lack of understanding and knowledge of women's biology has had cruel and damaging consequences when it comes to pregnancy and childbirth.

Although miscarriage is very common, we rarely talk about it openly, leaving women to endure it quietly and alone, often convinced that something they did may have caused it. Without solid data about the impact of drugs, both prescription and nonprescription, on a fetus, pregnant women's consumption is highly regulated and restricted, which can feel infantilizing and oppressive. An incomplete understanding of female anatomy, including the organs, muscles, and fascial involved in childbirth, have led to years of women suffering—unnecessarily—from postpartum incontinence and pain.

Instead, the void is filled with opinions and information from sources that are not always accurate and often rooted in particular value systems. They frequently leave women feeling confused, alone, afraid, or, worse, ashamed. As a result, our culture has adopted the belief that sacrifice and suffering—in silence—are simply the costs of becoming a mother.

When my daughter was an infant, I worked as the staff food writer at a newspaper in Seattle. A large part of my job was asking questions and finding experts who could answer those questions. Fueled by the urgency of new motherhood, I decided to apply my work habits to what was now my other full-time job: mother. I found an evolutionary biologist who studied human milk, set up a Skype date, and asked her all my questions about breast milk.

What I learned astonished me—not just the biological facts about the substance that my body was producing but also that there was so much more data available about breast milk, and research being conducted on it, than I ever would have known. The information gave me a new admiration for my body—and it felt to me like information that should be common knowledge. So I turned what I learned in that interview, along with my own experience with breast-feeding, into an article—one intended to celebrate a beautiful biological process as well as advocate for more support for new mothers.

To my surprise, the article went viral. Its success helped me see that it wasn't just me who was desperate for this sort of information—there were many of us. In an era of rapid screen scrolling and short attention spans, it turned out thousands of people across the world—and not just breast-feeding moms—wanted to read thousands of words about science, women's bodies, and motherhood. They wanted to share the piece with their friends and families, to engage in spirited debates and conversations about it.

As I continued seeking answers (I had *many* more questions about subjects beyond breast milk), I learned that we are currently awash in fresh knowledge about pregnant bodies: How the placenta develops and how important the organ is to our overall health. How the perceived risks of drugs and alcohol reflect public health policies more than the findings of the latest research. How the difficulty and length of labor can be dramatically reduced with something so simple as the constant support of another human being. And how the cells of our children, whether we carry them to term or not, live on in our bodies for a lifetime.

The more I learned what was *not* in the pregnancy guides I'd read, the more I knew this was knowledge that could not only inform women but also help to mitigate our fears and anxiety. In a culture in which our bodies are routinely scrutinized, and often criticized, these discoveries felt to me like hope: information that might put us in awe of our physical forms, even hold us in a profound, celebratory embrace.

Unfortunately, much of this emerging science remains largely out of the reach of the over four million people who give birth in the United States each year. It can take decades for knowledge to trickle down—through updated academic textbooks, medical school curricula, a new generation of health-care providers—finally to us, the people who need this information the most. This lack of knowledge impacts our health and bodily freedom.

When we don't know and appreciate our bodies—when we feel disconnected from their inherent cycles and rhythms—our power, rights, and choices are more easily taken away from us. This disembodiment is part of what makes it possible for a male elected official in 2016—without shame, second thought, or consequence—to say of pregnant women, "I understand that they feel like it is their body. I feel like it is separate—what I call them is, is you're a host."[3]

Control over our own bodies is an essential freedom, but it's one women have never been able to take for granted. We live in a society that, even as it relies on us to exist, continually conspires to remove us from our bodies and to punish us when we exercise our rights to—or not to—reproduce. True female reproductive health, which is the foundation of everyone's health, requires that the social systems in which we live allow us to make informed choices about what is best for each of us.

Science is an ongoing, imperfect process and its scope is far from complete. For centuries, the territory of human biology was limited mostly to the bodies of white men. Science has taken us this far but must continue to evolve and respond to people's real-time experiences in order to serve all of us. In the meantime, we have each other—communities of women and parents, telling our stories, holding each other up with our shared experiences. I picture them as spiderwebs strung up throughout the world—an infinite, if sometimes invisible, network of strength.

This book is not meant to be a traditional pregnancy guidebook with advice on what or how to do things. It's intended to be a resource rooted in emerging science and real-life stories. Its lines of inquiry follow my own experiences and curiosity, which are wide-ranging but by no means complete. I'm not an expert. When I started working on this book, I was mostly a tired and desperate new mom with a long list of questions. The stakes have always felt high and deeply personal; it's precisely what has motivated me. In research and writing, I've learned a lot—and it hasn't always been comfortable. As I've heard from and spoken with many different people about their own journeys, I've had to confront my own biases and assumptions. Looking back on the article that led to the opportunity to write this book, I realize that the ease I had with breast-feeding created a blind spot about just how hard it can be for others. How the pressure, intentional or not, that we place on new mothers—not just to breast-feed but to enjoy pregnancy, to give birth a certain way, to "bounce back," to be happy—is unnecessarily stressful and harmful.

This book is subtitled "A Feminist Journey Through the Science and Culture of Pregnancy." Women in America have been denied power and agency for so long that, as many of us benefit from the gains made by the work of the feminist movement, it can be hard to remember how many of us haven't yet gotten the same opportunities. Forty years ago, when I was born, mainstream feminism didn't necessarily take into consideration the concerns of my mother, an immigrant from the Philippines with three young children who worked full-time. As with so many other subjects, most dominant discussions, scientific studies, and representations of pregnancy do very little to acknowledge the incredible range of experiences. I wonder if the title and language of this book, which rely on the gendered term "mother," will feel out-of-date as our understanding of who gets to experience pregnancy and birth, as well as our views of gender, continue to evolve.

We need to keep telling our stories, but we also have to learn to listen. Our stories—and the diversity of our perspectives—are invaluable.

No book on pregnancy can or should offer an ideal model of it, because there is no one correct way to become a mother. If pregnancy and motherhood have taught me anything, it's that I have zero interest in judging people or the choices they make. What matters to me is that we have real choices—and the information to get there.

We owe it to ourselves to learn, to demand science and evidence, to seek out the full spectrum of information as it exists now. As much as I've learned from the experts that I've interviewed, though, I've learned just as much, if not more, from my "mom friends," as well as the acquaintances and strangers who have generously shared their stories with me. Their commitment to parenting every day, to giving over their bodies, whether they feel like it or not, breeds its own hard-won wisdom.

And so we should insist, too, that medical professionals and scientists listen to us, the people on the front lines having the babies. Our bodies are telling us stories and giving us new clues and information every day.

"We are volcanoes," wrote the American novelist, essayist, and poet Ursula K. Le Guin. "When we women offer our experience as our truth, as human truth, all the maps change. There are new mountains."

My hope in writing this book is the same as Le Guin's: "That's what I want—to hear you erupting."[4]

ONE of YOU

CHAPTER 1

NOW WHAT?

When, for the first few weeks, the only evidence of pregnancy I had was the memory of my doctor's voice on the phone and a plastic stick that I had peed on, it was hard to know what to do with myself. Freshly pregnant, but also fresh from the sadness of losing a pregnancy, I found myself asking the same question over and over: "Now what?"

Try as I might, after learning that a microscopic proto-person was growing inside me, I wasn't able to just go about living my life as usual. I had a hard time simply "being" pregnant, and I felt compelled to "do" it properly. I knew that I wanted to do everything I could to keep myself and my baby healthy, learn about the risks involved, prepare for the physical changes to come, and try to stay positive and hopeful. I knew I should also do my best to make the most of the time my husband and I had left as a family of two.

"Sometimes birth choices are not about perfection or fears but just the way we happen to be living," wrote Randi Hutter Epstein in her cultural history of childbirth, *Get Me Out*.[1]

I think the same is true for the choices we make throughout pregnancy. The way we happen to be living right now is marked by an overwhelming amount of information, as well as an astonishing number of ways to get that information. It can add up to a lot of mental noise.

Yes, we get facts and guidelines from our doctors, midwives, and nurses, but we only see these care providers every few weeks and, typically, for less than thirty minutes per visit. There's a lot more time—and questions, big and small—that make up the daily experience of pregnancy. And so, increasingly, we turn to websites, books, online forums, and social media. There is no shortage of pregnancy advice out there, and all of it can be summoned to our screens in a matter of seconds.

Quick searches on common topics such as contractions, early pregnancy symptoms, and birth options yield pages of answers from a seemingly infinite variety of websites including Web MD, Healthline, Mother Rising, The Bump, BabyCenter, BabyCentre UK (in case you want to see what moms in other countries are told), What to Expect, Parenting, Giving Birth With Confidence, Momtastic, Babble, *New York* magazine's The Cut, American Pregnancy Association, MedicineNet, Fit Pregnancy, Cafe Mom, the Mayo Clinic, Women's Health, Planned Parenthood, Mama Natural, Huffington Post, and the National Institutes of Health.

These resources represent a mix of medical organizations, personal blogs, health and lifestyle magazines, scientific research, feminist publications, health-care providers, news organizations, and government institutions. They each serve a particular agenda, but it's hard to tell whose exactly. The authors of these articles, lists, and summaries (if they are even listed) don't always link to sources, so it's hard to trace where the facts are actually coming from.

In a mere ten minutes of scrolling through my Facebook feed, these articles all showed up as suggested or sponsored posts, or as content from websites that several of my friends had "Liked":

6 Strange Things Your Body Will Do While Breast-Feeding

What I Wish I'd Known Before Giving Birth: 4 Things About Pregnancy One Mother and Yoga Teacher Learned the Hard Way

8 Crucial Things Men Need to Know About Pregnancy

23 Underrated Parenting Products That Actually Work

7 Co-Sleeping Myths That Are Actually True

Every article we click on through Facebook and Twitter, every Google query we type in, and every Instagram post we "Like" triggers algorithms, so the information and images we see are constantly being custom-fitted to our interests—and our fears. The messages, which come quickly, one after the other, tell us to trust doctors but also to be skeptical. To trust birth and be open to its unpredictability, but also be scared because you might die. They say it is okay to let your baby cry it out at night, she won't remember in the morning, but also be aware that her body will be flooded with the stress hormone cortisol and her unconscious will learn that you, her mother, are willing to abandon her when she needs you the most.

When pregnant friends ask me for advice about things, I tell them, only half-jokingly, to never look on the Internet, because you can find whatever answer it is you are looking for. Want to know that home birth is empowering and orgasmic? No problem. Want to learn how home birth is fatal and the midwives who encourage it are inept? Check. Want to know that sitting in a hot tub for ten minutes will help your tense, pregnant body relax and feel better? Got it. Want to read about how it could dangerously raise your core temperature and that you probably shouldn't risk it? Click right here. Sifting through these contradictory messages amplifies the already tremendous sense of responsibility you have as an expectant mother—not only do you have to take care of yourself and the helpless embryo inside you, but you need to sort through all the information and figure out The Truth.

Several friends recommended *The Healthy Pregnancy Book*, written by husband-and-wife medical team William and Martha Sears. (The Searses are the authors of a series of books, the Sears Parenting Library, which includes *The Baby Book*, *The Baby Sleep Book*, *The Breastfeeding Book*, *The Fussy Baby Book*, and *The Discipline Book*.) William is a pediatrician and medical professor and Martha is a registered nurse; together they raised eight children. I figured I could learn a great deal from them.

Indeed, I did learn from the Searses. But when I first opened *The Healthy Pregnancy Book* and began reading the introduction, I was startled by an image. There on the second page was a gray, delicately shaded pencil illustration of a baby nestled cozily in a womb, its arms and legs crossed. A thought bubble emanated from the baby, carrying a firm message: "Mama, take good care of yourself so I can grow better."

The illustration appeared regularly throughout the book, offering pointers and seeming to suggest that I needed help with my priorities. "Mama, make our health your hobby," the baby reminded me on page 4. I was only eight weeks pregnant (my fetus was kidney bean–size and arguably had more in common with a bean than a person), and yet here was this fully formed baby admonishing me for mistakes I was already making.

"Do you really want to eat that?" the baby asked incredulously on page 54. It was reclining next to a red box titled, "Science Says: Gain Extra Weight, Labor Extra Long."

Pregnancy guidebooks like these are valuable—they offer a basic understanding of the biological process of pregnancy, fetal development, and childbirth—but my experience with so many of them was that they were more instructive and prescriptive than informative. I don't mean to pick on the Searses here—other books such as *What to Expect When You're Expecting* and *Your Pregnancy Week by Week* were just as loaded with value judgments, some subtle, others brazen. Chapter six of *The New Pregnancy Bible: The Experts' Guide to Pregnancy and Early Parenthood*, the most easily available guide at my public library, is titled "Looking Great" and suggests that pregnancy is a good time to "pay special attention to your hair, skin, teeth, breasts, and feet."

If you want to know what to expect, it is that a lot of people will have a lot of expectations about your pregnancy and what you "should" be doing. And these expectations can break you.

But, I wondered with each book I picked up and put down, instead of focusing on what is "good" and what is "bad" in the external world of pregnancy, why don't we invest more time and resources in understanding what is going on in its vast, internal world? Women deserve to have access to information so we can make our own educated choices—not information repackaged in the form of instructions about what those choices should be.

Instead of learning how to care for my nails or make a pregnancy salad, I wanted to learn about the placenta, the entirely new organ that my body was growing—the one that was making it possible for me to nourish and sustain my daughter with just my blood. I wanted to know what causes one pregnancy to make it to term and what causes one to end prematurely. I wanted to understand why the onset of labor and the course of birth, which happens to thousands of people every day, is so painful and unpredictable. These things seemed like pretty basic stuff.

There is plenty of useful information out there, but there is just as much targeted content and marketing material that influences not just how we feel about pregnancy but how we feel about ourselves. So many sources instruct us on what we ought to do—and how: how to arrange our priorities, how to move and what to eat, how to think about emotional fulfillment.

In pregnancy, I thought a lot about the women who came before me. My own mother willingly endured three C-sections.

She didn't use any pregnancy books, didn't have the Internet, and never lost hours of her life down the rabbit hole of Baby-Center forums. She loved my brothers and me fiercely but didn't know a thing about the term "attachment parenting." I thought of Lola Lily, my maternal grandmother, who lost two babies and birthed nine others in the Philippines and never had a single ultrasound. She was a professor of chemistry, an avid ballroom dancer, and a charmingly vain woman. It wasn't hard to picture the horrified expression that would come across her face if I mentioned taking a break from dyeing my gray hair for fear of the (possible) negative effects on my fetus.

Many of us, without thinking, will pick up our phone to Google something before we use it to call our own mothers or friends. We've been trained to discount informal experience in favor of more official, definitive resources—even when the origins of these things are dubious or unclear. Advice and information now comes less often from average people who are giving birth and rearing children and more often from medical professionals, online influencers, and so-called experts.

*

Women have always grown, birthed, and raised babies with the benefit of knowledge passed down through generations of other women. For centuries, in every culture around the world, midwives guided birth. They were mothers, grandmothers, aunts, and neighbors—older women who had no formal training other than decades of firsthand knowledge and experience. They advised laboring women on when to move, rest, or push, offered physical and herbal comfort, delivered babies, and tended to mothers and newborns in the days and weeks after birth. They understood pregnancy and birth as significant but normal events in the lives of women, not illnesses or conditions that needed to be treated.

But in late nineteenth- and early twentieth-century America, against the backdrop of a rapidly industrializing and increasingly wealthy nation, a new expert—the doctor—came to be the indispensable authority on these topics. In his 1894 book *The Care and Feeding of Children,* Dr. Luther Emmett Holt advised against relying on women's wisdom and experience, warning that "instinct and maternal love are too often assumed to be a sufficient guide for a mother."[2] His words paved the way for physicians to set the rules mothers would be expected to follow.

The 1910 publication of *Medical Education in the United States and Canada* by Abraham Flexner, a review of medical schools across the country commissioned by the Carnegie Foundation, led to millions of dollars in funding for schools such as Harvard, which enrolled mostly upper-class white male students. This money came from the charitable foundations of wealthy industrial families such as the Carnegies and Rockefellers. With considerably less resources, most smaller schools, including medical schools that enrolled black and female students, were unable to compete and were forced to close.[3] Medicine moved from a healing art practiced by various types of people in different classes to a profession requiring eight years of expensive training.

At the time, nearly half of all babies born in America were

delivered by midwives, most of them working-class immigrants and black women.[4] This figure was deemed unacceptable by members of the emerging gynecological and obstetrical community. In 1912, J. Whitridge Williams, a professor of obstetrics at Johns Hopkins University, set out to promote his formally educated peers over lay midwives. For his report "Medical Education and the Midwife Problem in the United States," Williams surveyed the faculties at 120 medical schools offering four-year courses in obstetrics. His results were surprising.

Williams found that many professors felt both unprepared to teach obstetrics and unqualified to deal with obstetrical emergencies. One man, who lectured on the subject, confessed that he had never actually attended a live birth. Instead of conceding that doctors might have something to learn from midwives, Williams doubled down on his agenda, insisting that the profession be eradicated. Midwives were dangerous. Doctors, he reasoned, would gain sufficient experience . . . eventually.[5]

In the years after, states passed laws requiring that babies be delivered by a licensed medical doctor and banning the practice of lay midwifery. Especially impacted by these new regulations were granny midwives, African American women who had, for generations, attended the births of babies of all races throughout the South. These women were less likely to be literate, less likely to be formally educated, and, because they lived and worked in rural areas, less likely to have access to the registration offices that would allow them to continue working legally.

The clinical expertise that physicians ultimately acquired often came at the expense of women—black women in particular. Dr. J. Marion Sims, a nineteenth-century Alabama surgeon, is referred to as the "father of modern gynecology." Sims created what would become the modern-day speculum, the duck bill–shaped tool that is familiar to anyone who has had a vaginal exam. He is most well-known for developing a surgical technique for repairing vaginal fistulas, tears or openings that form between the vagina and urinary tract or anus, causing fluid and feces to involuntarily leak out of the vagina. At the time, fistulas were common after childbirth and were embarrassing and disruptive to people's lives.

Sims developed his technique through years of surgical experimentation performed exclusively on a dozen enslaved women, without the use of anesthesia. Their owners brought these women to Sims, only three of whom—Anarcha, Betsey, and Lucy—were named in his records. Slaves were considered property and, as such, the women were never paid for their participation. Only after mastering his technique (he operated on Anarcha thirteen times) did Sims repair the fistulas of white women, all with anesthesia.[6]

During the early twentieth century, women weren't just driven out of the field of health care, they were also actively excluded from accessing medical education. And with that, the responsibility of caring for pregnant women shifted to men. Women today, even though they comprise the majority of health-care workers, do so in roles that are mainly subservient to men, who disproportionately occupy positions as physicians and hospital administrators. It's not a coincidence.

But women still play the most crucial role in the business of pregnancy and childbirth. We make and have the babies, which means we still get to call more than a few shots.

In the early 1900s, wanting to avoid painful childbirth experiences overseen by men, women demanded to be sedated with drugs during delivery. They insisted it was their right to have peaceful and, in some cases, entirely unconscious births. Pain-free childbirth became a feminist cause. The American medical community quickly moved to give mothers what they wanted: births using Twilight Sleep, a drug and method developed by German physicians. Unfortunately, in their rush, doctors failed to administer Twilight Sleep under the same meticulous protocols, which led to traumatic births. The movement lost momentum. But the desire for pain relief remained, and other drugs were developed and used for decades. Until the 1970s, many women gave birth under the influence of tranquilizers and anesthesia. After that, the feminist cause became reclaiming birth from drug-induced hazes and the hands of male doctors. American women increasingly wanted to be conscious for the full experience of birth. Today, feminism means supporting women in whatever method of birth that they want.

The medicalization of pregnancy and birth marked a huge change—one of many that have filled the last century. Hutter Epstein summarizes a few of them like this: "Obstetricians went from placing a stethoscope on the belly to listen for the pitter-patter of a heartbeat to using ultrasonography to snap a 3-D image of the fetal heart. Birth went from home to hospital, from drug-free to drugs on delivery, from midwives to doctors, from the occasional C-section to C-sections on demand."[7] Pregnancy, once an ordinary part of a woman's life, is now a medical condition that requires supervision by experts. Prenatal care—amniocentesis, cell-free DNA testing, limitations on substances we ingest—are all relatively new, modern concepts.

There is no single approach to pregnancy and childbirth that is best. While the origins of American obstetrics and gynecology may be infuriating, many of us have benefitted from it. Advancements in the field have improved health outcomes for mothers and babies. And, for better or worse, this is the medical system under which most of us receive our prenatal, maternity, and postpartum care. Where we are now—balancing contradictory views on pregnancy along with a deluge of all too accessible contradictory information about it—is, again, a reflection of how we happen to be living right now.

So where do we go from here? How we live now is destined to continue evolving, to change. It already is.

Demand for information is not going to go away. As technology improves, we're only going to be able to see better images of our fetuses, and earlier and earlier. There will be even less mystery. Having information about pregnancy also feels more useful than ever because—and I can't believe I have to write this in 2018—we women still don't have full legal control over our bodies.

Today women in America can be criminally charged for poor, and often tragic, outcomes of their pregnancies.[8] In some states a mother can be charged with chemical endangerment of her child if she exposed it to controlled substances in utero, even if the drugs or medications were intended to protect her fetus from greater harm—and even if the child is born healthy.[9] You can have your baby taken away for making what others deem to be the "wrong" choices about child care.[10] In this sense, it feels irresponsible not to be informed about every possible substance you consume and every possible circumstance that could occur during pregnancy and your child's infancy.

For all the talk of "empowered birth," in American society mothers and expectant mothers have far less power than we should. Everything we do is measured against an impossible standard of what we ought to do, what is "best." Variation is seen not simply for what it is, biological and cultural variety, but as a deviation from what is perceived as normal.

I believe we all want to make the conversations around pregnancy and motherhood as inclusive and encouraging as possible. But because we don't all receive the support we deserve, we often find ourselves dividing along arbitrary lines about the choices we make: what we drink (or don't drink) during pregnancy, how we give birth, how we feed our kids, where we let them sleep, and so on. While all of these things are important in day-to-day life, they are not the problems or issues that have kept American women down for centuries.

The vast majority of resources on pregnancy and motherhood direct our eyes and minds to issues that don't actually matter in the grand scheme of things. The problems we face are much bigger: a culture in which men hold nearly all of the legal and economic power; a society in which whiteness is considered the norm and superior to other races and cultures;

an economic system that relies on, but does not adequately value, domestic work that is performed overwhelmingly by women (or, if you prefer: patriarchy, white supremacy, and American capitalism). It's not what many people want to hear, but it is our reality: there aren't any easy answers to questions about pregnancy—they are all political. To deny this is a luxury we can't afford.

I read dozens of books on pregnancy and motherhood, and with each one, I was aware that I was not reading them with all parts of myself. I placed my body in one box, my brain in another. I divorced my mind from the story of my own life. Women of color, lesbian and queer people, as well as people who do not fall within a gender binary, understand that our full personhood or womanhood is still considered conditional. We know that the "normal" or "average pregnant" person discussed in books does not refer to us. In doing research, studies I've read break down data by race and ethnicity. Numerous times, I found myself, a Filipina woman, lumped into the category of "Other."

A. K. Summers's graphic novel *Pregnant Butch: Nine Long Months Spent in Drag* was the first book about pregnancy that I was able to bring my full self to. Our stories were very different, but the emotional undercurrent was the same. Though Summers was eager to grow her family, her pregnancy required that she give up the hard-won comfort it took her years to find within her body as a masculine-presenting, butch lesbian.

By the end of Summers's pregnancy, the physical transformations left her feeling alien from her body. "I am not myself," she declares as she floats upside down on a black page in a puffy space suit, tethered to a spaceship far in the distance. "I am tears and I am snot. I am anemic and I am purple veins. I am boobies."[11]

I've spent my entire nonpregnant adult life in a body with large brown breasts, a soft, round belly, and plenty of curves—a body I have struggled to see as beautiful, and sometimes even acceptable, in a culture that overwhelmingly celebrates people who are thin and white. Yet I saw my own leaky, weary self in her drawing: disoriented and alone, fumbling my way through a strange galaxy with so many swollen parts.

If we quit putting stock in the idea that pregnant people are doing things either well or poorly, we could speak the truth: that we are all just doing the best with what we have. When it comes down to it, we are all left with the same thing: our bodies. And they are astounding, in both their uniformity and infinite variety.

Pregnancy is a time of rapid change. So many things are happening inside our bodies all the time, and our physical form and the way we feel seem to change daily. Our minds are constantly churning with new thoughts, processing new emotions. And yet, as women who have lived in our bodies for decades before we began sharing them with someone else, pregnancy can feel not like something we are living but instead something that is happening *to* us: something about which everyone else has an opinion—a story, a set of values, expectations—that they can affix to our condition and that has little to do with who we actually are as individuals.

The tidy tales of reproduction that we repeat over and over (a mommy and a daddy get together, the egg and sperm join, then—voilà!—nine months later, there's a baby) belie the complex process through which we conceive and grow our young, not to mention the reality of what parenthood looks like today. While commercials for home pregnancy tests still offer the same predictable scene—a young, overjoyed woman, tears running down her cheeks, emerges from the bathroom and falls into the loving and outstretched arms of her husband—the picture has changed for many of us. It is the rare and fortunate person whose journey to pregnancy and motherhood has not involved some, and sometimes years of, struggle.

Is there any other process as complex as pregnancy that has been wrested into such an oversimplified, one-dimensional narrative? As the years pass, so many things about human reproduction change and expand: the reach of technology, the age at which women become mothers, the way we arrive at pregnancy, our ideas about traditional gender roles, gender itself, and the language we use to talk about it, as well as our concept of what constitutes a family.

According to the Society for Assisted Reproductive Technology, 65,175 babies conceived through in vitro fertilization (IVF)—a process by which eggs are harvested and sperm are collected, and insemination takes place in a petri dish—were born in the United States in 2015. Even as the American birth rate has declined over the last decade, the rate of IVF has steadily increased.

"There is no longer one dominant family form in the U.S.," a 2015 Pew Research Center report found. "Parents today are raising their children against a backdrop of increasingly diverse and, for many, constantly evolving family forms."[12]

The latest edition of *What to Expect When You're Expecting* declares that a family, no matter what its makeup, is a family. "But," it states, "as you read . . . you'll notice references to traditional family relationships. These references definitely aren't meant to exclude expectant moms (and their families) who don't mold neatly into that traditional family form. Please mentally edit out any phrase that doesn't fit and replace it with one that's right for you and your loving family."[13]

Our resources have yet to catch up to our reality, putting the onus on their audience—the audience they should be serving—to adjust to outdated information.

For all the information out there, we still have no idea how complex pregnancy will be until we are living it. We have no idea how contractions will actually feel, and no one ever tells us how much our bodies accomplish through the pain contractions cause. Women go into childbirth unaware of physical realities of delivering a placenta, of recovering from a C-section, and of the possible physical implications of birth. We hear almost nothing about the emotional landscape of the postpartum experience: the alienation from your own body, the massive identity shift.

Knowledge and authority about pregnancy and birth—which make up our individual and collective histories and guarantee our future—shouldn't be held exclusively by people with certificates, degrees, or high-profile publishing platforms. It should be something that all women talk about openly and have access to, without cost.

We are all born from female bodies, and so we have all experienced birth firsthand. We were all female once, too.

All humans will grow female parts unless, around the tenth week of pregnancy, hormones called androgens direct a fetus to develop testes and a penis. Female is our origin sex.

Growing and birthing a child is an experience as individual as it is universal. The more we are told there is a "right" way to do it, the stranger—and lonelier—it can be. And the journey to motherhood, which draws you deep into your own body, all the while preparing you to prioritize another person ahead of yourself, is already fundamentally isolating. For all the physical changes of pregnancy, eventually that baby leaves your body, stretching and scarring and altering it on its way out. The squishy ball of soft skin that was once inextricable from yours will gain the strength to crawl, then walk, away from you. You are left with yourself—someone familiar yet totally different.

Looking back on all those hours I spent on the Internet and reading books, I don't actually remember many details from the flood of information that continually washed over me. What I do remember is the counsel I got from one of my best friends, Elizabeth.

Elizabeth always answered my random pregnancy questions, texts, and calls. Despite taking an eight-week class in preparation for childbirth, I realize that it was my friend's description of her first labor that offered me the best glimpse of what was in store. She said she knew it was time to go to the hospital when, down on all fours in her bedroom, she "roared like a lioness." It was a phrase that, until I heard my fairly reserved and modest friend say it, I was quite sure I would never hear her say.

Elizabeth sent me a box of odds and ends left over from her two pregnancies: packets of tea, lotion for my belly, and, notably, twenty individually wrapped pregnancy tests left over from an online bulk order. I never actually used all of those tests, but now they are the items that strike me the most in their kindness: a reassurance from someone who had also been through loss that there was room for my fear and anxiety in pregnancy—that it was okay to be scared. It was a conversation we had silently, each of us on opposite ends of the country, but it was a clear message that stays with me to this day, one I want to share with others.

There is no right or wrong way to be pregnant, to become a mother, to make a family. There is only one way—your way, which will inevitably be filled with tears, mistakes, doubt, but also joy, relief, triumph, and love.

Women have been speculated about, experimented with, and reported on for years, but rarely have we been given the chance to simply tell our own stories, to own our undeniable authority. These are the conversations we should be having. Let's start a new one now.

CHAPTER 2

IMPERFECT CHOICES

There is a pleasure in holding on to the secret of pregnancy, even with all its early uncertainty and excitement. For a few hours or days, nobody but you (or you and your partner) know. To be alone with your body, with a quiet sense of all the potential and power that it holds, and just an inkling of all that lies ahead, is an intense, and intensely private, thing. But it doesn't last long.

Soon enough, your body will give you away. You begin to protrude, to change into a public entity. To the world, your changing shape signals that you are a pregnant person first and yourself second. You become a repository for other people's hastily blurted thoughts, a blank screen for them to project their hopes, fears, beliefs, and instructions.

It's not all bad—I smile every time I think of the woman who, while giving me a gel manicure, found the two thickest copies of *In Style* magazine in the salon and dramatically draped them over my belly to protect it from the UV rays of the drying lamp. But, as the fellow pregnant woman I once stood next to in a coffee shop as we waited for our lattes said as she pointed to her belly, "Too many strangers have too many unsolicited opinions about this thing."

Our culture tends to think about pregnancy in terms of the limitations it places on our bodies and lives, big and small. No matter what your personal style might have been before you got pregnant, when you go shopping for maternity clothes, you are likely to find little more than stretchy shirred-on-the-sides cotton tops (often striped) and empire-waisted dresses. When you sit down at a restaurant, a well-intentioned server will automatically remove the wineglass at your place setting. As you carry bags of groceries out of the store, perhaps balancing one atop your belly, a man passing by won't offer to help you, but he will ask, "Whoa, you sure you should be doing that?"

For centuries, in the absence of science and reason, women's bodies—especially our bodies as reproductive vessels—were subjected to wild speculation and morality, usually at the whims and desires of men. We're still subject to these things today.

The birth position favored by most doctors—*lithotomy*, meaning flat on your back, knees flexed, feet in stirrups—is a far cry from traditional, more active squatting and kneeling positions portrayed in the art of ancient Greek, Egyptian, Persian, and Aztec cultures. Lying on the back didn't become the preferred position until the seventeenth century, when French king Louis XIV, a bit of a voyeur who enjoyed watching childbirth from behind a curtain, commissioned the construction of a special viewing table so he could get the best angle possible.[1]

The "husband stitch," a colloquial term used by US obstetricians, is an extra stitch that was sometimes sewn into a woman after her perineum was torn or cut, via episiotomy, during childbirth. The purpose of the unnecessary extra stitch was to make the vaginal opening smaller and tighter than it was before birth in order to increase a husband's sexual pleasure.[2]

It was only in the twentieth century that researchers came to understand menstruation as part of our species-sustaining reproductive process and not a hideous scourge that caused food to spoil. Before this revelation, people relied on information from sources like the Bible, which, in Leviticus 15:19, says: "Whenever a woman has her menstrual period, she will be ceremonially unclean for seven days." Roman historian Pliny the Elder wrote: "Contact with [menstrual blood] turns new wine sour, crops touched by it become barren, grafts die, seeds in gardens are dried up, the fruit of trees falls off, the bright surface of mirrors in which it is merely reflected is dimmed, the edge of steel and the gleam of ivory are dulled, hives of bees die, even bronze and iron are at once seized by rust, and a horrible smell fills the air."[3]

That may sound antiquated and superstitious, but as recently as 1977, a leading medical journal, the *Lancet*, published a letter speculating that flowers held by menstruating women would wilt as the result of "menotoxin," an invisible, nefarious substance secreted through the pores of women who happen to be on their period.[4] (To be clear: It's a myth. There is no such thing as menotoxin, or "menstruation poison," and there never was.)

In 1970, a junior high school teacher in Cleveland named
Jo Carol LaFleur was placed on mandatory maternity leave
during her second trimester because her supervisors were
concerned that "her pregnant body would alternately disgust,
concern, fascinate, and embarrass her students."[5] At the time,
many school districts had either no maternity leave policy
or put teachers on forced leaves determined entirely by administrators. LaFleur filed suit and, in the case of *Cleveland
Board of Education v. LaFleur,* the Supreme Court ruled that
LaFleur's constitutional rights had been violated. The decision gave women legal protection, allowing them to pursue
both their career and family goals without fear of repercus-
sion or losing their jobs. This was in 1974.

Perhaps the darkest side of pregnancy is being routinely
infantilized by people who offer their advice and opinions
on how to be the best possible host/incubator for your baby.
They include coworkers, supervisors, family, strangers, the
medical community, even the government.

In both meaningful and banal ways, we condescend to pregnant women, treating them like children who need guidance,
help, and protection. There are many rules. Eat nutritiously but
not too much. No soft cheeses, deli meat, or raw fish. ("What
do women in Japan do?" I always wondered. Turns out they
keep eating sushi.) Beware of coffee. Exercise, but don't elevate
your heart rate too much. And of course, steer clear of alcohol
or drugs (even the prescription kind that you might need to
function on a daily basis).

Individuals arrive at pregnancy with habits, weaknesses,
familial triggers, illnesses, predilections—the human baggage

we are born with and accumulate over the course of a life-time. Would-be mothers are no more or less virtuous than any other person, but our expectations for them immediately shift when pregnancy enters the picture.

The strictest, most high-profile limitation we place on pregnant women is abstinence from alcohol. And with good reason: alcohol is the only drug that is cytotoxic or terato-genic, meaning it can kill or damage cells. If a mother con-sumes excessive amounts of alcohol over a prolonged period of time, we know that her baby may be born with fetal alco-hol syndrome (FAS), a condition that can include physical deformities and delayed brain development.

Because of this risk American women are advised, per federal mandate, to avoid all alcohol during pregnancy. Al-though our culture is thoroughly soaked in alcohol and its presence in our everyday lives is ubiquitous (whether you partake or not), our policy on consuming it in pregnancy is zero-tolerance. Unfortunately, these guidelines fail to take into account the very recent context out of which they grew.

The term "fetal alcohol syndrome" was coined in 1973 by two researchers at the University of Washington. In the thou-sands of years preceding, few people questioned or worried about its effects on a fetus. Alcohol was even administered in-travenously to women as an attempt to delay preterm labor.[6] How, in less than five decades, did we arrive at a point where alcohol, widely tolerated for centuries, became pregnancy's number one prohibited substance?

"When it came to preventing fetal alcohol syndrome, pol-itics played a role, as well as science," writes historian Janet

Lynne Golden in her book *Message in a Bottle: The Making of Fetal Alcohol Syndrome.*[7] The women's liberation movement of the 1960s meant that in the 1970s, equality—including the new understanding that women were just as susceptible as men to alcoholism—was a major cultural current. At the same time, the Nixon administration was beginning its "war on drugs" and new streams of federal funding were made available to study the effects of drugs on health.

The 1970s were also a time of growing interest in the fetus. Technology made it possible to actually see them—tiny beings with wee noses, fingers, and toes—on ultrasound screens. Doctors were able to draw fluid through amniocentesis to diagnose illness in utero. And the effects of thalidomide, an antinausea medication given to many pregnant women that unknowingly led to babies being born with stunted limbs and missing digits in the 1960s, were also fresh in people's minds. These helpless little beings captured our collective imagination and lawmakers began to operate under the idea that all fetuses needed protection. Fetal health became more of a concern than maternal health.

In 1977, public health officials suggested that expectant mothers have no more than two alcoholic beverages a day. FAS affected only infants whose mothers were severe alcoholics, but because there was no clear, scientifically determined "safe" amount of alcohol, a blanket public health approach that warned all pregnant women to avoid drinking gained traction. By 1981, the surgeon general issued an official instruction for pregnant women and women *considering* becoming pregnant "not to drink alcoholic beverages."

All women—whether they drank occasionally, abstained from it entirely, or abused it regularly—received the same guidelines. Instead of investing in counseling, social services, and prenatal care to help the smaller population of alcoholic women who were actually at risk of giving birth to children with FAS, federal institutions instead chose to offer a public health mandate that offered high-risk women the same resources and attention as mothers with little to no risk.

Unsurprisingly, it was not an effective strategy. (As Dr. Jim Walsh, a Seattle-based family medicine doctor who specializes in addiction issues, told me, "Telling an alcoholic not to drink is probably the worst thing you can do. The whole point is that they can't stop.") Even after an extensive public campaign to spread the message of the dangers of drinking while pregnant, rates of FAS did not decline. According to Golden, "the syndrome ultimately became a marker of maternal misbehavior rather than an indication that new measures were needed to help alcoholic women."[8]

Instead of reconsidering its approach, the government doubled down on its strategy, adding warning labels to the alcoholic beverages that line the shelves of grocery, convenience, and liquor stores. This messaging, revisited and upheld by the Department of Health and Human Services in both 1990 and 1995, is still in place today.

Since then, warnings about alcohol use for women—and not just pregnant women—have arguably become more extreme. In 2016, the Centers for Disease Control and Prevention released an educational flyer for health-care professionals titled "Drinking Too Much Can Have Many Risks for Women."

While the design of the poster was modern, the message was tinged with old-fashioned paternalism.

Listed among the risks of drinking for pregnant women and their fetuses were "miscarriage, stillbirth, prematurity, fetal alcohol spectrum disorders, and sudden infant death syndrome." And the risks for *any* woman who drinks? "Injuries/violence, heart disease, cancer, sexually transmitted diseases, fertility problems, unintended pregnancy." It is, apparently, every woman's job to avoid pregnancy, sexual assault, and sexually transmitted disease. By not drinking.[9]

The poster makes clear the belief that women are creatures that need the expert guidance of medical professionals to navigate the world: "Providers can help women avoid drinking too much, including avoiding alcohol during pregnancy, in 5 steps."

When I was pregnant with my daughter, I got together regularly with my friend Abbie, who was due a few months ahead of me. We'd go for walks and have dinner and, usually, a drink. While planning a date when Abbie was eight months pregnant, I began suggesting a few restaurants. She cut me off.

"Actually, do you just want to come over?" she asked. "I really want to have a beer, but I'm too big to drink in public anymore. People look at me weird, or they say something, and I just can't deal."

How many pregnant women have hidden out in their homes, fearing judgment from others who can't handle them making decisions about their own bodies?

We know for certain that excessive amounts of alcohol can lead to cellular damage and, in some cases, fetal alcohol syndrome. The difficulty is that we have no collective definition for what "excessive" means. For some women, based on their metabolism, three drinks will be too much. For others, the number might be five. But one beer every now and then is unlikely to do any harm.

The science is difficult to parse because there are ethical limitations to conducting tests on pregnant women. You can't force them to guzzle martinis or glasses of wine to study the potentially damaging effects. As such, many studies are based on self-reported data, sometimes years after pregnancy. This methodology inherently leads to recollection bias and inaccuracy. The design of studies may also mistakenly group women with very different drinking habits into the same category. There might be a group of women who have "four drinks a week" but no distinct categories such as "four drinks in one night" and "one drink on four different nights." Not only are these scenarios remarkably different, but the quantity of alcohol consumed in one session has different effects on the fetus. And then there is the fact that FAS is not a guarantee: despite a mother's heavy alcohol consumption, some babies are born perfectly healthy.

Dr. Jim Walsh mentioned cases of women who gave birth to fraternal twins—one with FAS, the other healthy.[10] "They were exposed to the same alcohol, obviously," he explained, "but there's a randomness to it. There's risk and then there's also bad luck."

Walsh oversees a clinic for mothers with addictive disorders that provides maternity care, as well as group counseling. The clinic, which he believes may be the only one of its kind in the United States, accepts walk-in patients dealing with chemical dependency issues at any stage of pregnancy.

The feelings Walsh described in his patients—the desire to do what is best for the baby, a longing to maintain their sense of selves, and, perhaps most of all, a tremendous fear of being judged—rang all too familiar. I'm not trying to minimize the complex issues that come with the combination of addiction and pregnancy, but the emotions all expecting mothers deal with are similar. The constant admonishing—the ever-growing list of "shouldn'ts" and "shoulds," the desire to be seen as "good" and "correct," is stressful for people dealing with addiction. It is also the dominant experience of being pregnant and a new mother in America.

Emily Oster, author of *Expecting Better: How to Fight the Pregnancy Establishment with Facts*, wrote that, when she was pregnant, she was frustrated by the seemingly endless, arbitrary, and often contradictory rules she found about consuming substances. She used her training as a data-driven economist to examine the studies cited as evidence for these rules. In many cases, she found that such guidelines are based on what she describes as "overinterpretation of flawed studies."[11]

Oster's conclusions about the quantities of alcohol and caffeine that can be consumed safely in pregnancy—a couple of drinks a week in the first trimester, up to one a day in the second and third; three to four eight-ounce cups of coffee a day throughout pregnancy—are much less restrictive. Her book, published in 2013, sparked a lot of conversation. It is part of a growing number of evidence-based pregnancy resources that look critically at widely accepted data and advice, and advocate for informed, personal decision making.

I'm not suggesting you make a choice with which you're fundamentally uncomfortable. Maybe you don't mind giving up coffee and you've never had a cocktail in your life. Maybe giving up raw tuna or soft, fudgy cheeses is a bigger challenge for you. Individuals value different things differently. My point is that the real question we should be asking expecting mothers is, "What level of risk are you comfortable with?"

Some people are willing to bend "the rules" as long as things fall within a low-risk zone. Other people find the restrictions of pregnancy reassuring. Rules offer us a semblance of control at a time when so much in our lives is chaotic. Rules also help us maintain the belief that, as mothers, we are responsible for the outcome of a pregnancy—if we make all the right choices, our baby will be perfect. Following rules helps us believe that we are eliminating as much risk as possible, which can be incredibly important, especially for people who have struggled to get pregnant or who have lost pregnancies.

But most of us also invite nuance into other areas of our lives—we make decisions based on what is best for ourselves and our families, balancing work and personal time, individual desires versus the needs of a group. We take the advice of our doctor or dentist and do our best to stick to it—flossing, if not every day, at least every few days, trying to eat less late-night pizza, and getting exercise when we can.

But when it comes to pregnancy, we can't seem to tolerate it, in part because messages we receive over and over are free of nuance, free of discussion. The weight of the responsibility is intense. This is often the first time in our lives that our choices physically impact the well-being of another human being. That is sobering. It makes us crave simplicity in a state of being that is inherently complex. I don't blame anyone for wanting certainty, but the truth is that there is little. Pregnancy is our first lesson in this surrender and submission. Eventually, our experiences—with pregnancy loss, labor, birth, and motherhood—will reinforce to us that there is little we actually control.

In pregnancy, developing babies are of the utmost importance, yes. But so are mothers. There are no babies without us. Without being allowed our autonomy—ownership of who we are, messiness, flaws, contradictions, and all—we can begin to fade into the background, a shadow to ourselves and our future children.

Pregnancy drew me inward. It forced me to consider not only my shifting physical form and the tiny person growing in my uterus but also to take stock of my desires and weaknesses.

Like many people, I had a good time in my twenties—maybe a little too good. I partied a lot, played faster and looser with rules, had a lot of fun, and stayed up late making connections with people that fuel me to this day. I lived right up to the edge of what I was capable of; it seemed the only way to be alive. Even though I was thirty-six when I got pregnant, I started feeling as though maybe that time wasn't so far behind me.

I became attached to a fantasy that Abbie and I concocted. We pledged that one day after our babies were born, we would have a blowout party night. Maybe New Year's Eve. We'd get babysitters or leave our husbands at home. We would drink and dance and party all night. I carried the thought around with me like a stone I picked up at the beach and absent-mindedly left in my jacket pocket, rubbing it between my fingers, delighting in its smoothness whenever I happened to remember that it was there. While existing in a highly regulated state of being, I relished the dream of rebelling against it all. I got caught up in nostalgia for a person that I used to be.

In pregnancy I didn't quite know who I was or who I was becoming. One thing I knew, though, was that I didn't want to lose myself.

*

When it comes to pregnancy and mental health, for many years the well-being of women—who are affected by depression at rates twice as high as men—was also devalued in favor of the fetus. For the millions of women prescribed antidepressants, mood stabilizers, and SSRIs (selective serotonin-reuptake inhibitors, which include the medications Zoloft, Lexapro, and Prozac), those who wanted to become mothers were told to wean off these medications in preparation for pregnancy. If they became pregnant while on medication, it was suggested that they cease taking it as soon as possible.

The effects of SSRIs on fetuses have been studied more than any other drug. While they do not cause a statistically significant risk of birth defects, they are linked to an increase in the risk of miscarriage, low birth weight, and preterm birth. But are these adverse effects on babies caused by pharmaceuticals, or are they the result of stress and events that mark the lives of mothers who have forgone their medication?

As in the case of alcohol, research on the effects of these drugs is limited because researchers can't conduct blind experiments on pregnant people. Unable to give half of their subjects a drug, the other half a placebo, and observe what happens, as they would do with the general population, researchers instead conduct observational studies between women who chose not to take medication during pregnancy and those who did.

Until 2015, the Food and Drug Administration used the risk classifications A, B, C, D, and X for prescription drugs in pregnancy. They indicated the range of negative effects, with A being "No risk in controlled human studies" and X being "Contraindicated in pregnancy."

When my friend Ann got pregnant in her twenties, over fifteen years ago, she was taking Zoloft (pregnancy category risk C: "Cannot be ruled out").

"My doctor told me, 'We don't really know the risks, but you should probably come off it,'" she said. "So I did. But then I had a miscarriage. And then my godson died. I got back on the antidepressants."

Distraught after her loss, at one point Ann confessed to her doctor her fear that a glass of wine she drank early in her pregnancy may have contributed to the miscarriage, even though logically she knew that wasn't the cause.

"It was my neuroses that really needed to be told that I was not to blame," she said. Instead her doctor asked her, "Why did you do that?"

She was devastated—and infuriated—by that response. "I was already scared of the medical establishment anyway," she said. "I felt incredibly dehumanized."

The drugs that Ann resumed taking made it possible for her to work through her grief, achieve professional success, and establish a secure partnership. She was in a good place when she got pregnant again.

The medical landscape had also changed since her first pregnancy. In 2010, researchers from Johns Hopkins University and the University of North Carolina urged physicians to have more nuanced conversations with their patients about antidepressant use in pregnancy so that patients could make informed decisions.

"The decision to use antidepressant medication during pregnancy or lactation must be weighed against the risks of untreated maternal depression and this risk/benefit ratio must be carefully discussed with each patient," they wrote. "Avoiding antidepressant use during pregnancy or lactation is often not an option."[12]

In 2015, the FDA replaced its risk classification system with a broader Pregnancy and Lactation Labeling Rule, which lists all available information on the effects of drugs on pregnancy and nursing infants.[13] Since many antidepressants seem to be relatively low-risk to fetuses and breast-fed babies, some doctors now let patients choose what they want to do. But the counseling and advice you get still depends heavily on who your doctor is.

For her second pregnancy, Ann knew that she did not want to stop taking her antidepressants because she was certain it would be best for her and, ultimately, her son. She invested a lot of time in finding a doctor who had experience dealing with issues that affected her life—depression, eating disorders, and infant death.

"Those of us who have had miscarriages, or dealt with infertility or other issues—we are not outliers," she said. "Many of us come to pregnancy with a lot of emotional involvement already and I don't feel like that gets discussed by your average ob-gyn. I needed to make sure that my doctor was going to be cool with all my stuff."

Ann said that being in her early forties—over a decade older and having lived through difficult life events since her first pregnancy—strengthened her resolve to find a doctor who really listened to her and cared about her health.

"I was much pickier the second time," she said. "And [my doctor] listened to me and said, 'No, you don't need to go off your medication. You don't need to put yourself through that.' And I stayed on it and it was fine."

More physicians like Ann's are insisting that we fully consider mothers' health needs—both before and after birth.

"I prefer to think that I'm really treating a system and trying to mitigate outcomes for the whole system," Elizabeth Fitelson, a psychiatrist at Columbia University Medical Center who specializes in women's health, told the *New York Times*. "That means you have to pay attention to a mom's capacity not just to bear a child but to take care of a child."

Fitelson estimated that about 10 percent of her patients could safely go off medication and that another 20 percent need to stay on it. And for the remaining 70 percent?

"It's a venture into the unknowable."[14]

As for as the possible effects of antidepressants on her son, Ann had this perspective: "Honestly, I don't even know what the long-term effects are on myself. Only that it helps me live."

Depression and anxiety are treatable illnesses—illnesses that can predate pregnancy or, just like preeclampsia or gestational diabetes, develop during it. Mental health issues continue after pregnancy as well. We know that 80 percent of new mothers report a range of mood changes, many of which pass in time. But as many as one in seven mothers will experience postpartum depression, a more serious condition that will not abate on its own and requires treatment.[15] Postpartum anxiety, though we hear less about it, may actually be more common than depression.[16]

Another mother I know, Lauren, has dealt with anxiety since she was in high school. She said that while it can be hard, it is manageable. Her anxiety usually flares up during life changes, so it wasn't surprising that she felt it during pregnancy.

But, she said, "I never experienced anxiety like I did when I had a baby. That was another level."

At her six-week postpartum appointment, Lauren's obstetrician asked her if she felt depressed.

"I told her, 'No, I don't have that,'" she said. "But she did not ask about anxiety at all, she did not ask if I had any thoughts that scared me. Meanwhile, the first five months, I had anxiety that grew and grew and [within six months] had taken over my life and my brain completely."

Lauren's postpartum anxiety developed into depression and, eventually, the rare disorder of postpartum psychosis. She experienced intrusive thoughts, became suicidal, and ended up spending several weeks in a psychiatric hospital. She is now in recovery.

Postpartum mood disorders are highly individual conditions. Symptoms include sadness, irritability, and fear, but also range from overeating to lack of appetite, from insomnia to oversleeping. Although experience with one or more of these conditions is quite common, it often makes new mothers feel alone. This isolation is compounded by the unrelenting job of caring for a newborn in its first months of life, a time when people are more housebound and also likely to ignore their own health in order to focus on their child.

Whether we are suffering from a clinically diagnosable mood disorder or the more common "baby blues," there is also a reluctance to show our true selves to others. We are emotional and hormonal messes; it is a fact of postpartum life. There is a biological underpinning to these mood swings, but new mothers are also under tremendous pressure to be happy (after all, we just had a baby!). We want to seem like we are holding it all together.

"After I left the hospital for the first time, I went to my doctor and put on a smile and lied about how much better I was doing," said Lauren. "The doctor bought it and said he was glad. After I left his office I got in my car and I wondered if there was a way to sneak off and kill myself."

As a society, we tend to mark mental illness, just as we do addiction, with stigma, as a character flaw. In Lauren's experience, mental disorders weren't things people talked about openly, and this contributed to the severity of her illness as well as a delay in her getting treatment.

"Before I recovered, I wouldn't have wanted people to know what I was experiencing because I didn't want them to label me as unstable, crazy, weird, etc.," Lauren said. "Sometimes I get the sense that I am more comfortable talking about it than some people are hearing about it."

*

The choices we make in pregnancy—how to balance the health of our babies with our own well-being—are imperfect ones. But we all have to make them. Because these decisions, and pregnancy itself, are marked with uncertainty, they can lead to feelings of tremendous insecurity. When things are unknowable, we have to use our imagination. In pregnancy, often our worst insecurities and fears are indulged, making a fraught state even more difficult. It makes us, a group of individuals each with the right to our own choices, the right to our own mental and physical health, feel alone. We are not.

Throughout pregnancy, I liked to lie in bed and imagine all the changes happening inside me: cells splitting, fingernails and eyelashes growing, veins spreading, brain and gray matter forming and folding. At times, these images fed my fears. I wanted everything to proceed smoothly, correctly—I worried that how I lived, who I was, could prohibit this from happening as it should.

But I tried my best, too, to let my imagination comfort me,

to open me. I relied on it to transport me into my old body, my body to come, other bodies, other experiences. Pregnancy connects you to so many people—past, present, and future—who have gone and will go through the same disorienting process. I tried to be as generous with myself as I would be to others. I'd tell myself that there was only so much that I could do to help this growing being along, only so much of myself that I needed to give up or change.

Pregnancy isn't just a reason to stop doing something. It can be a reason to start something else, to grow. To surprise yourself. I would suggest that the forty or so weeks of pregnancy are not a time for women to arrest their own development or put themselves in a holding pattern. It is, by nature, a state of constant transformation and change. The nausea and exhaustion of one trimester gives way to the energy and bawdiness of the next, the discomfort but profound pride and satisfaction of the last. We are always in flux, always a work in progress.

One evening last summer, I found myself on the front porch at a friend's party, talking to a new mom. We've known each other for years, and although we've never been close, we've spent many late, fun nights together with friends. We reminisced a bit about those times and got to talking about postpartum life, life with her daughter. She seemed really happy, and I told her so.

I am, she replied, and then, unexpectedly, she went on to tell me that for several years before she got pregnant, she had been doing drugs, amphetamines mostly, pretty much every day. I was both surprised and not, and impressed by her honesty. She had wanted to stop for a long time but had never known how. But when she found out she was pregnant, the idea of quitting was no longer hard.

"It helped me get my life together," she said.

Pregnancy—even the long-term possibility of it—can be highly motivating. According to a report published by the CDC, over 20 percent of women who smoked in their first or second trimester quit by the third. Those who continued reported smoking fewer cigarettes as their pregnancies progressed.[17]

"Becoming a mother was the most transforming thing in my life," a woman named Drora Kemp wrote in response to a *New York Times* article about the complex psychological process of becoming a mother.[18] "It made me, a party girl, a smoker and drinker, into a person with a mission—raise my son the best way I could."

I could relate. The person I was in my twenties was long gone. Over the course of a decade, in incremental shifts that I never noticed, I had already said good-bye to her. In pregnancy, I had invited someone else besides my daughter into my body. Instead of fighting her, I let her take me along, like a friend pulling at my hand, leading, whispering in my ear that she would never leave me behind.

CHAPTER 3

AN ORGAN AS TWO-FACED AS TIME

In early pregnancy, I found myself obsessively thinking about my placenta, the organ growing inside my body and nourishing my baby. Let me say that again: the entirely new *organ* that I was growing, alongside another human being, inside my uterus.

I wanted to know everything about it and how it functioned. My basic understanding was that the umbilical cord, and by extension the placenta, somehow helped feed the baby. I read my pregnancy books, scanning them for information, looking up "placenta" in the index. There was plenty of acknowledgment of the placenta's existence but not much insight into what exactly it does. The brief description of the placenta in BabyCenter's *Pregnancy: From Preconception to Birth* seemed to exist mainly to scare me: "Through the placenta, your baby is exposed to what you take into your body, so make sure it's good for both of you."[1]

For many years the placenta was commonly referred to as afterbirth, which tells you exactly how we've regarded it: as an afterthought. Yes, the placenta is delivered after the baby is delivered, but it's the organ that precedes the second set of organs growing in your body.

Because we don't often pay it the attention it's due, most of us don't know that at any given moment, 20 percent of our blood is traveling through the placenta, keeping our future child or children nourished. We don't hear about its remarkable immunity work, fighting off and eliminating pathogens while also allowing antibodies that exist in a mother's body to pass through and on to the baby. It is a forcible barrier, but not unyielding. It allows protective proteins into the fetal environment, and also allows fetal cells to cross into the mother's body, where they may take up residency for decades.

Along with the most fundamental structures of the body, the placenta is built in the first few weeks of pregnancy. By the end of the first trimester, it has established its crucial, direct connection with the maternal blood supply. My first trimester was marked by a level of exhaustion like I had never experienced before: a pure, bone-deep tiredness that would send me, if I sat down to rest for just a moment, into a comatose, blackout, sleep-of-the-dead-type sleep. Upon waking, for just a split second, I'd have no idea where I was or what day it was. After learning about the placenta, it all made sense: I wasn't just building a whole person out of nothing but also a fairly hefty new organ that was siphoning off my blood supply.

Nourishing a fetus is just one of the placenta's many jobs. It's also responsible for gas exchange (swapping oxygen for carbon dioxide), eliminating waste, regulating the baby's temperature, helping fight potential infections, and building immunity. It acts as part of both mother and child's endocrine systems, producing hormones that support pregnancy and fetal growth, and even one that helps signal the onset of labor. The organ is a workhorse, doing the duty of the fetus's kidneys, heart, and lungs before they exist.

By the end of a pregnancy, a placenta may weigh up to two pounds. It is formidable. Unfurled and laid out flat, its tissue would cover up to 150 square feet—about the size of the average office worker's cubicle. After delivering the organ, many women, if given the opportunity to look at it, are shocked by its considerable size.

One of my best friends, Rivka, who has birthed two children and two placentas vaginally, lamented that no doctor, midwife, or childbirth instructor had adequately prepared her for the physical reality of delivering it. "No one told me that after I finally pushed the baby out, I'd still be having contractions and needing to push this whole other thing out. So just know that," she told me as my due date approached.

Just weeks before our conversation, when I was seven months pregnant, I read an article in the *New York Times* about some of the newly discovered biology of the placenta. This was a few days after I had taken my gestational diabetes test, a sadistic procedure that involves chugging a bottle of a syrupy sweet "glucose tolerance beverage" (I chose the fruit punch flavor) and sitting in a waiting room for an hour as the sugar coursed through my veins and made my heart race.

As I sat there, jittery and sweaty, the baby did somersaults in my womb, and my belly surged and distended under my stretchy gray cotton maternity dress. I was disturbed—and also intrigued—by how quickly the glucose seemed to have made its way through my bloodstream and placenta.

The article explained how, unlike the placentas of most other animals, which establish fairly superficial connections to the uterine wall, the human placenta goes deep, infiltrating up to one hundred uterine arteries, and growing thirty-two miles of capillaries.[2] (Compare this to both our small and large intestines, which, if uncoiled and laid out, would only be about twenty-five feet long.) How the placenta goes about doing this is both incredible and harrowing.

But there was something else, too: the language used by the reporter, Denise Grady, was so vivid. As a writer, I recognized it as the enthusiasm you catch when you encounter an especially inspiring subject or person.

> The front line of the invasion is a cell called a trophoblast, from the outer layer of the embryo. Early in pregnancy, these cells multiply explosively and stream out like a column of soldiers. They shove other cells out of the way and destroy them with digestive enzymes or secrete substances that induce the cells to kill themselves.

Among the experts Grady had interviewed was Dr. Susan Fisher, a professor of obstetrics, gynecology, and reproductive sciences at the University of California–San Francisco. Fisher oversees her own lab, the Fisher Lab, where she and her team of researchers were among the first to discover the highly invasive nature of the placenta, as well as the specific molecules it uses to do its work.

"When I first read this anatomy, I couldn't believe the whole world wasn't studying this," Fisher said. "Compared to what we should know, we know nothing."

I found myself nodding in agreement, enraptured. I wanted her to tell me more.

Two years later, I spoke with Dr. Fisher on the phone. Through the course of our hour-long conversation, she began many of her sentences by saying, "The other really interesting thing about the placenta is . . ." Her enthusiasm for the organ is contagious—enough to convince you that the alphabet posters in kindergarten classrooms should declare that "P is for placenta," rather than trivial things like peas, pencils, or penguins.

Explaining more about how trophoblasts penetrate the uterine wall—and are allowed to do so by the native cells—Fisher said, "They do this remarkable thing that no other cell normally does: they start making molecules that identify themselves to the mother's body as being a blood vessel cell rather than a placental cell. They're such chameleons, it's amazing."

In the years since Fisher first observed this invasion process, other researchers have found that only certain cancer cells, including breast cancer cells, engage in this sort of vascular mimicry. Her discovery has opened up new channels for approaching and studying how cancer grows in the body.

Our understanding of this organ may also hold the key to improving the outcomes of people who undergo organ transplants. The placenta does not, technically, belong to the mother. Our bodies may create it, but it is part of the developing child, which means it is also made up of 50 percent genetic material from the father. The organ—and the fetus—are both foreign to the mother's body, yet she tolerates them, even allowing the placenta to take hold of and scramble her body's structures.

When an organ is transplanted into a human body, the natural inclination of the recipient's body is to reject it. It is only through aggressive suppression of the immune system with drugs that the organ may be accepted. Fisher and other scientists are investigating how the placenta convinces a mother's immune system to accept itself and the fetus. If we can understand how it prevents her body from rejecting them, we may be able to better understand how to prevent organ rejection in transplant patients.

When Fisher first started her study of the placenta, she was staring at cells through a microscope—they were immobile, fixed to a slide. She could only look at sets of isolated cells during different stages to see what they did over time. But she and her team made a major breakthrough by getting cells to develop, in real time, in the laboratory, allowing researchers to spy on the processes that normally happen deep inside a mother's body. This has enabled scientists to ask further questions about their function, and what molecules are involved.

According to the National Institute of Child Health and Human Development (NICHD), the placenta is "the least understood human organ and arguably one of the more important, not only for the health of a woman and her fetus during pregnancy but also for the lifelong health of both." In 2015, the NICHD launched the Human Placenta Project, and has been directing funds to research efforts to better understand the organ throughout all stages of development and pregnancy.

A healthy placenta is directly tied to a healthy pregnancy. If the organ cannot properly develop or establish a connection to the uterus and blood supply, that pregnancy will likely be lost. Placental abnormalities such as placenta previa, in which the placenta attaches low in the uterus and covers the cervix; placenta accreta, in which the entire placenta or parts of the organ penetrate too deeply into the uterine wall and cannot detach after birth; and preeclampsia, in which the organ's blood vessels do not form properly, leading to high blood pressure and dangerous conditions late in pregnancy, can cause difficult and frightening births, even maternal death.

"We now know that placental function determines the outcome of pregnancy," said Fisher. "And how pregnancy goes is a large determinant of adult health."

In 1990, British epidemiologist David Barker hypothesized that a fetus's environment has profound and long-lasting effects on his or her health. Barker's theory was supported by data linking higher rates of cardiovascular disease in certain adults to both low birth weights and mothers' malnutrition during pregnancy. It was especially apparent in children born to women who experienced famine and extreme food rationing in Europe during World War II. Prenatal or in utero "programming," as Barker termed it, also left people more susceptible to heart disease and type 2 diabetes.

"The womb may be more important than the home," Barker wrote.[3]

In the decades since Barker published his findings, other researchers have expanded his theory to include conditions such as allergies, obesity, osteoporosis, and vision problems. Other studies have shown that women who experience common pregnancy complications such as gestational diabetes and high blood pressure (both of which may affect and be affected by the placenta) are at a greater risk for cardiovascular disease later in life.

Cardiovascular disease and type 2 diabetes are two of the deadliest and most common chronic illnesses in the United States. We should be concerned about not only the placenta's role in pregnancy but also its role in drawing up the blueprints of adult health, as well as the health of mothers. And yet the placenta, though it is integral to the health of all human beings, is only regarded as a footnote in the study of women's reproductive health, which, along with women's general health, is consistently undervalued in American society.

Up until very recently, government-funded research has been conducted almost exclusively by, on, and for white men. It was only in 1993 that Congress passed the National Institutes of Health Revitalization Act, a law requiring that women and minorities be included in clinical trials funded by the federal government's National Institutes of Health. 1993. Two and a half decades later, women are still underrepresented in medical research. While heart disease is the leading cause of death among women in the United States, for example, less than one-third of cardiovascular clinical trial subjects are female.

The placenta is also difficult to study. Its life span is finite; it reaches maturity around thirty-four weeks, after which it begins aging. It exists in service of the fetus and, when a fetus is born, its tour of duty is over. Though it plays a crucial, life-sustaining role, it doesn't stay in the body for a lifetime. It must come out.

And when it does come out, the placenta is at another disadvantage: it's arguably less visually appealing than an organ like the liver, which, despite its strong, ferrous smell, is uniformly dark and smooth. The liver has a certain gothic beauty. A placenta has two sides—each grisly and wholly distinct.

The maternal side of the placenta, which alters and fuses to the strong, muscular wall of the uterus, is made of pulpy red blobs. After detaching from the home it carved out for itself, it looks appropriately meaty, like a juicy, raw pot roast. It is as shimmering and bloody as a fresh wound. The fetal side teems and crawls with thick scarlet and blue veins and arteries. It's a gnarly tangle of bound and naked blood vessels. It's a carnal version of satellite photos of river deltas—small and large tributaries, all reaching from remote corners to fill the powerful stream that is the umbilical cord. The cord, which is made of one vein and two arteries surrounded by a gooey substance called Wharton's jelly, is encased in a thick white membrane called amnion. It's the fetus's lifeline, connecting the placenta to the baby's abdomen, where, after birth, the fleshy, wrinkled circle we call our belly button remains for a lifetime, the only evidence of this profound physical relationship.

Susan Fisher believes that the placenta's complex structure is part of the reason we know so little about it.

"It has a structure that is very, very hard for a lot of people, even professionals, to understand," she said.

Fisher is a frequent speaker at conferences and gatherings of obstetricians, gynecologists, and reproductive workers.

"After I go through my initial spiel on the basic structure of the placenta—and these are rooms filled with professionals—I will have a line of people coming up to talk to me. And the gist of what every person says is: 'Really? This really happens?'"

Fisher laughed and then grew quiet. "If health professionals don't understand this, they're certainly not going to try to explain it to their patients."

And so pregnant people don't hear much about their placentas. We hear virtually nothing about this hybrid interface tethered to two people, keeping them separate but connected. We don't hear about this remarkable organ that is the site of the first communication and cooperation between mother and child, but also their first conflicts and negotiations. We fail to understand how this conduit connects the present, past, and future, and how its influence can be felt through all these places in time.

*

Far from the confines of laboratories and hospitals, most mammals—including domesticated dogs and cats, wild lions and monkeys—eat their placentas immediately after giving birth. Even animals whose diet consists only of leaves and fruits engage in this practice, called placentophagy. Every day throughout the animal world, mothers are eating their placentas. Human beings are a rare exception. The organ is considered medical waste that is typically discarded and incinerated.

While people do not widely ingest the placenta, it does enjoy a revered place in many non-Western cultures around the globe. For the Hmong people of Southeast Asia, the word "placenta" is translated as "jacket" and viewed as a being's original clothing. Traditionally, the placenta was buried under the birthplace, most often the home. After death, the Hmong believe that a soul returns home, where it must retrieve its placental jacket in order to ascend and be reunited with its ancestors. Without a coat, a soul is doomed to wander for eternity, cold and alone.

Among other cultures, including Native Hawaiians and the Mossi people of Burkina Faso, the placenta is valued as a vital part of a baby's passage into the world. It is ceremonially buried or placed back into nature, with the belief that it will strengthen the child's connection to his or her home and ancestors. Dried placenta has been used for centuries in traditional Chinese medicine to treat liver and kidney issues.

Over the last few decades, a growing number of American women have begun embracing—and ingesting—their placentas, including celebrities like Kim Kardashian. (In a small survey of 189 women who consumed their placentas, researchers found that the overwhelming majority of them were white, wealthy, and married.)[4] While women today aren't necessarily eating them, raw and feral, there has been an increase in placental encapsulation, the process of putting them into easily digestible pill form. Proponents of placenta encapsulation claim that consumption will help the uterus contract and heal more quickly, make breast milk more abundant, and help to prevent postpartum depression.

When I was pregnant, I was curious enough about encapsulation to look into it. When I saw that birth workers charged an average of $250 for the service, though, I decided it wasn't that important to me. But toward the end of my pregnancy my doula, Sage—the woman my husband and I hired to support us through labor and delivery—asked me if I was interested in having her do it. Because she was still learning, she was willing to do it for free. I accepted.

Sage and I had worked together briefly at a bookstore a few years back. We spent a lot of time behind the counter talking about food, particularly the African American food she grew up with in Texas and the Filipino food I was raised on. She was tough-minded and smart. She was also a single mother who, when her son was very young, weathered breast cancer and a double mastectomy. I knew Sage had an understanding of the many ways things can go easily or difficultly in life, and a determination to thrive in all of it. At some point along the way, in addition to studying traditional herbal medicine, she had started doing birth work. As someone who grew up never being treated by a doctor or nurse who looked like me or knew much about my family's culture, it was important to me that my doula be a woman of color. I trusted Sage implicitly and wanted her by my side.

Because my daughter was delivered via Cesarean section, I never actually saw my placenta. But Sage did—and she became intimately acquainted with it. Before labor, I authorized the hospital to release my medical waste to her. After surgery, they double-bagged it in thick blue plastic bags and gave it to her. Around midnight on a Friday night, two hours after my daughter was born, Sage put my placenta in her purse and walked the mile back to her apartment, where she put it in her refrigerator before falling into a deep sleep. (I had been in labor for over twenty-four hours, so she was pretty tired.)

The next morning, she took it out and washed it in her kitchen sink.

"Placenta has a very specific smell. It's like liver," she told me when I asked her for all the details. "Your placenta was very big—maybe the size of a vinyl record, and between one and a half to two inches thick. It was beautiful."

To be honest, I half expected Sage to express some mild level of distaste or repulsion at handling one of my organs. But she was unfazed, running through her process with the clarity and reassurance of any good recipe.

Traditional Chinese medicine views labor and birth as a process that leaves the body with empty space, which is considered yin, or cold. Following these principles, Sage aimed to promote my recovery by adding yang, heat and energy.

"I took my Dutch oven, lined it with fresh ginger, lemons, and sliced jalapeños, and steamed it lightly. It shrank, darkened, and hardened liked cooked meat," she said. "Because it is cooked meat."

When it was done, it had acquired a uniform grayish brown color. She sliced it and dried the pieces in her circular food dehydrator, where they become porous and brittle.

"And then I put it in a coffee grinder and made it into

a powder," she said. "My kitchen smelled like I had been cooking innards or organ meat, that really earthy smell that I love."

A few days after my daughter was born, Sage came to our house with a brown glass bottle filled with pills made of our placenta. I took eight pills a day for the first couple of weeks, and then tapered off, eventually stopping before I finished its contents.

I was an exhausted physical wreck before I started taking the capsules, and I felt that way for a good month. Taking them didn't make me feel much different, but I also had no idea how I was supposed to be feeling. I was without a map. I did not experience postpartum depression, though I did cry multiple times each day and sometimes couldn't bring myself to get out of bed for hours at a time.

So did my placenta pills work?

I don't know. Currently there is no proof that taking placenta pills will accelerate postpartum recovery or offer new mothers any other benefits. In fact, according to a study published in 2015 by researchers at the Northwestern University School of Medicine who analyzed empirical human and animal studies of placentophagy, "there is no scientific evidence examining its effects in humans, and the data from animals are inconclusive."[5]

There are also no standards for the production of placenta pills or regulations about what goes in them. It can be done in the home, but increasingly, encapsulation services include sending the placenta to an outside facility for dehydration and encapsulation. In 2016, a newborn in Oregon who was having difficulty breathing was diagnosed as having group B streptococcus infection, and the bacteria were found in the placenta capsules that the mother had taken after delivery. (Every pregnant woman is screened for group B strep in late pregnancy, but in this mother's case, the test had been negative and the infection was later determined to be "late-onset.") Researchers in Oregon who investigated the incident concluded that "the placenta encapsulation process does not per se eradicate infectious pathogens; thus, placenta capsule ingestion should be avoided."[6] The risk of this individual case spurred the CDC to include the local researchers' warning in one of its weekly national newsletters.

The most compelling evidence for placental encapsulation resides in the many stories of mothers who say that it helped them. As Sage told me, "I like proof. But I also like intuition, stories, and testimony."

Here in the Pacific Northwest, people of the Coos, Makah, Tillamook, and other tribes have been telling stories of great earthquakes. The accounts have been passed down through at least seven generations. A few decades ago, after centuries of believing this region to be geologically stable, seismologists found scientific proof that it is anything but. In her 2015 Pulitzer Prize–winning *New Yorker* story, "The Really Big One," Kathryn Schulz detailed the inevitable, large earthquake that could decimate much of the coastal Northwest. Schulz, as well as other scholars, noted that the facts scientists had only recently "discovered" have long been understood by indigenous peoples.[7] But their stories had been dismissed and ignored for centuries.

Just because science hasn't proven something doesn't mean people don't know it.

*

For hundreds of years, ancient Romans worshipped Janus, the god who presided over passageways and doors, beginnings and transitions. Because he looks to both the future and the past, he is portrayed as having two faces. A poet named Robert B. Shaw described Janus as being as "two-faced as time,"[8] which is how I have come to think of the placenta. It literally reaches back into our origins, mothers' bodies, while simultaneously making future generations possible.

Time is the ultimate frenemy. Just as it moves us forward, it also moves us away, slowly, from the people we have worked to become. We gain valuable things as time marches ahead— experience, knowledge, hopefully wisdom—but we lose things, too. For parents, it creates an ever-widening distance between us and our children. It allows them to grow, to turn their backs to us.

When Sage brought me the placenta pills, she also brought my baby's umbilical cord. She had no use for it, but it hadn't been her place to throw it away. Not knowing what to do with it, I stuck it in the freezer, where for two years it lived behind a bag of black, overripe bananas destined for a loaf of banana bread that never came to be.

After talking to Susan Fisher, I pulled the umbilical cord out of the freezer and set it on the counter to defrost. It was wrapped in plastic and stuck inside a ziplock bag. It looked like a giant blood clot and scared me a little. But as it sat on the counter, growing warm and supple, my feelings toward it softened as well.

Just like my daughter, it had been a part of my body. But unlike my daughter, a wild dynamic creature who hurls herself further into the world each day, always changing, the cord stays the same. It will never grow again.

The spring after my daughter was born, we planted a small magnolia tree by our house. A year later, the tree's first white blossoms appeared, and she raced to bury her nose in the flowers and inhale their strong perfume. Months later, on a sunny winter afternoon, my husband and I dug a hole in the cold ground while our daughter napped and buried the umbilical cord—this thing that is part me, part him, and part her—under the tree. We placed the fleshy ribbon through which so much of my blood had run into the dirt, to be part of our small place here on earth.

It gave us so much, I told him, maybe it has more to give.

CHAPTER 4

BEFORE I HAD A BABY, I HAD A MISCARRIAGE

Five years ago, six weeks into a wanted pregnancy, I woke up bleeding. Thick globs of blood and tangles of tissue dropped out of me, staining my inner thighs and clothing. I called a consulting nurse, who calmly walked me through a few questions. Bleeding is normal, she assured me, as I sat silently on the other end of the line, frantic, seething, and not believing a single word that came out of her mouth. I hated her. I hated my body for what felt like a betrayal.

It was November, and my husband and I had planned to tell our families about the pregnancy at Christmas.

The nurse told me to wait a few hours and, if I was still bleeding, to come in so they could draw my blood to check my hCG level. Human chorionic gonadotropin, or hCG, is a hormone that doubles every two to three days during early pregnancy.

That afternoon, the bleeding had become heavier. I went

in for the blood test. The next morning, my doctor called with the results, telling me that they were inconclusive and that I should probably come in for another test tomorrow to make sure that my level was dropping, and that I was in fact miscarrying. But I didn't need another test to tell me what I already knew.

It was a full week before I stopped bleeding. To me, what I was losing was matter, cells—not a baby. And yet the matter, for a couple of weeks, annihilated my rational mind. In just six weeks of pregnancy, nothing in my life had really changed. And yet, as it slipped and oozed out of me and I was powerless to stop it, it was replaced by a screaming sense of loss.

The only reason I didn't stay facedown on my floor for a day, or a month, was because my husband insisted that I go to work. He never tells me what to do (he's smarter than that), and that's probably the only reason I listened. Later, I asked him why he insisted I go to the restaurant that night and wait tables.

"Sometimes when people are really raw, the easiest way to get through the hardest part is to stay busy," he said. "It wasn't about not dealing with things—you knew what was happening—but reminding yourself that the world wasn't over. I wanted you to be able to get away from it for a little bit."

I worked that night, but as I walked the floor, smiling, serving steaks, busing tables, and opening bottles of wine, I could feel my own juices running out of my body. I couldn't get away from it that day, not physically, and not ever.

After I started telling people what had happened, many

of them told me not to worry. They pointed out that at least I now knew I could get pregnant. Over and over, I was told I could try again. For many women who have experienced pregnancy loss, healing becomes contingent on hope, on the promise of another pregnancy. But those directives, which come from well-meaning partners, friends, family members, and health-care practitioners, can get in the way of the more complex, healthier—and often slow—process of grieving and recovery.

For a few weeks, that embryo the size of a pea felt like an unfathomably large black hole into which, at moments, my sanity was at risk of being sucked. I didn't sleep well. I cried, seemingly all the time. I watched videos of Beyoncé talking about her miscarriage—"The saddest thing I've ever been through"—on YouTube over and over.

Instead of telling our families I was pregnant that Christmas, my husband and I did something else. We flew to Little Rock, Arkansas, on Christmas Day, rented a car, and drove to Memphis, where we spent a few days eating barbecue and fried chicken, and drinking bourbon. We paid $10 each at the door of a juke joint where the price of admission included a red Solo cup, allowing us to help ourselves to unlimited refills from a keg that sat on the floor, late into the night. We were sad, but we were drunk, and we talked loudly about the importance and beauty of our freedom.

The next day, we went to the National Civil Rights Museum at the Lorraine Motel, where we each stood in the exact spot where Dr. Martin Luther King Jr. was assassinated. In Arkansas, we hiked on the Trail of Tears, walking part of the route that members of the Choctaw, Cherokee, Muscogee, Seminole, and Chickasaw nations took, fighting disease and starvation after the US government forcibly removed them from their ancestral homelands.

We drove through Money, Mississippi, where, in 1955, fourteen-year-old Emmett Till was beaten, mutilated, and murdered, his body thrown into the Tallahatchie River, for talking to a white woman. In Jackson, the capital of Mississippi, I saw a family burning wood and trash in a drum on their front lawn. The windows of their house were broken; the fire was for heat. It was in that moment that I began to understand that while my loss was sad, it was not a preventable tragedy.

As we drove north back to Little Rock, I stared out the window as the landscape whirred by and repeated the lines of Elizabeth Bishop's poem "One Art" inside my head like an incantation: "So many things seem filled with the intent / to be lost that their loss is no disaster."

*

I have been pregnant—knowingly—four times in my life. Before I gave birth to my daughter at the end of 2014, I'd had a miscarriage in 2008, an abortion in 2009, and another miscarriage in 2013. Half of my pregnancies have ended in miscarriage. This might seem shocking, but it's actually quite ordinary.

According to a 2013 study by researchers at the Albert Einstein College of Medicine, most people believe that miscarriage is a rare occurrence that happens to only 5 percent of women.[1] In reality, miscarriage ends up to 20 percent of known pregnancies—roughly 750,000 to 1,000,000 every year in the United States. The true percentage is almost certainly higher considering the number of women who miscarry so early that they may never recognize the pregnancy as anything more than a late period.

Let's talk for a moment about the term "miscarriage." It's objectively terrible. Think of the words that begin with the same prefix: mistake, misstep, misplaced, misspelled. "Mis" seems to imply not only that something is wrong but that you have an active role in making it so. According to the Albert Einstein College of Medicine study, 40 percent of the women surveyed who experienced a miscarriage said they felt they had done something wrong to cause their miscarriage, and 47 percent expressed feeling guilty.

Scientists know that the majority of pregnancy losses are caused by aneuploidy—chromosomal abnormalities that, for reasons we don't totally understand, result in forms of life that are incapable of being carried to term. Fetuses with other chromosomal irregularities, such as Down syndrome and Klinefelter's syndrome, can still grow into healthy, full-term babies.

Yet the same survey found that the most commonly believed causes of miscarriages are things like stressful life events, lifting heavy objects, and having previously used a contraceptive intrauterine device (IUD). All of these "causes" suggest some responsibility on the part of women. And they all are unrelated to miscarriage.

There's a lot that scientists don't yet know about pregnancy loss. Most of the insights we have gained about miscarriage have not been the result of medical research dedicated to this topic. Instead, many discoveries came about as the by-product of work from scientists investigating things like chromosomal abnormalities and placentas. These researchers analyzed spontaneously aborted human fetuses and products of conception in part because they were in convenient, abundant supply. Why no one thought to study the reasons *why* they were in such supply is mind-boggling.

The clinical term for miscarriage is "spontaneous abortion," which feels, yes, clinical. For everyday life, I prefer the term "pregnancy loss," because that's exactly what it is. What exactly is lost, though, lies entirely in the heart and mind of each woman who experiences it.

*

Many people are uncomfortable talking about pregnancy loss, so they don't. And it's no wonder—any meaningful discussion of it requires acknowledging death, blood, tears, and items being expelled from the vagina.

The existing literature on pregnancy loss is largely dominated by stories of people who have been through multiple, consecutive losses ("recurrent pregnancy loss" is defined as three or more consecutive losses). Other, more scientific books strongly emphasize hope but don't always offer much insight into the "why" of loss. There are few resources for those of us who might have one loss or two. And we are in the majority—recurrent loss affects 1 to 2 percent of women.[2]

"[Recurrent pregnancy loss] is a tragedy," said Dr. Kristen Swanson, dean and professor at the College of Nursing at Seattle University. "But that's not the everyday version of miscarriage."

Swanson should know. She began studying pregnancy loss three decades ago as a doctoral student. Since then, she has interviewed and counseled hundreds of women about pregnancy loss and care. Swanson was also dean of the School of Nursing at the University of North Carolina, and, for more than twenty years, on the faculty of the University of Washington School of Nursing.

As a PhD student in the 1980s, Swanson, who had just given birth to her son, attended a support group for new mothers. On that particular day, the group hosted a guest speaker, an obstetrician who spoke about pregnancy loss.

"I listened like a nurse," she recalled, "because he was using words like 'spontaneous abortion,' 'products of conception,' 'diagnosis,' and 'prognosis'—medical terms."

Afterward, women in the group were eager to share their own experiences. Swanson was struck by the markedly different words the patients used: they spoke of loss, grief, babies, emotions, and mourning.

"There are two totally different languages used by practitioners and women who have experienced pregnancy loss," Swanson said. "My awareness happened in that moment. I knew this was something I could study."

At the time, Swanson found no published papers on the subject and no research tools with which to begin considering it. She decided to design and send out a survey to a few hundred women and write up the results. She asked women two questions about their losses: *What is it like? What made you feel cared for?*

"We should always take miscarriage as an absolutely normal life event," said Swanson. "It's a transition, part of living and dying. Every single day, your body is sloughing off fluids and cells that may be harmful to you. With miscarriage, you are entering a very natural process. The body is wise. It recognizes a pregnancy that could never be carried to term."

In the very early stages of pregnancy, the production of hormones—which act as chemical messengers throughout the body, sending various signals at various times—increases. In those first few weeks we are awash in a strange soup of estrogen and progesterone, which affect everything from the breasts to the bowels to the brain. (By frustratingly sudden turns, these hormones can make you feel exhausted, incredibly aroused, or nauseated.) When pregnancy loss occurs, those hormones suddenly rush away, and women may become swept up in a chemical ebb tide. The sadness and anxiety that follow may have intertwined physiological and emotional roots that are hard to detangle.

"The emotions that go with [miscarriage] can be huge," said Swanson.

Grief is complex and often feels overwhelming, but in most cases it lessens after three to four months. For women who have prior experience with depression, though, or who lack a support network, these feelings can deepen into anxiety and depression, and can linger for up to a year.[3]

Then comes the reckoning of what was lost, which is unique to each person and happens on its own timeline. The reactions to pregnancy loss are as diverse as the women who experience them—essentially infinite.

Informed by the results of her survey as well as in-person interviews with women, Swanson developed a model for caregivers in how to treat women experiencing pregnancy loss. Her model, the Theory of Caring, is based not on sympathy but empathy. Nurses treat and nurture their patients with a personal sense of responsibility. Her theory defines specific acts that health-care providers can perform: knowing, being with, doing for, enabling, and maintaining belief. According to Swanson, the most important message to offer a patient is that she can recover and work through pregnancy loss—not that she will, or will even want to, get pregnant again.

Though it was created specifically to care for women who had experienced pregnancy loss, Swanson's Theory of Caring has since been adopted as a model for general nursing and patient-driven care at hospitals around the country.

I wonder what else we might learn simply by listening to women.

*

The experience of pregnancy loss can be wildly divergent, even within one life.

My first miscarriage happened eight years ago, just days

after a doctor's appointment. My doctor at the time had asked me a routine question—the date of my last period. I couldn't quite remember, and then I realized it had been more than six weeks earlier.

She ordered a urine test; I was pregnant. I wandered out of the clinic and called a friend, who within minutes picked me up in a nearby IHOP parking lot. A few hours later, my boyfriend, who would later become my husband, picked me up at her apartment, where I had been sitting on the couch crying.

I—we—did not want to be pregnant.

Two days later I started bleeding. I went back to the doctor's office, where they performed an intrauterine ultrasound with a long wand. "There is nothing in there now," I remember someone saying. "You must have miscarried."

I didn't ask any questions. I don't remember feeling anything besides relief. My body had made an executive decision, and I felt grateful to it for that.

But five years later, when I was pregnant again and my husband and I were excitedly planning to tell our families at Christmas, the circumstances had changed. I still remember, on that morning when I began bleeding heavily, hanging up with the doctor and starting to walk the three feet from my bedroom to my bathroom and not getting all the way there. Instead, I lay down on the carpet in the hallway and sobbed for an hour.

A friend of mine, someone I used to work with, recalled a similar experience. She and her wife have been trying to get pregnant for more than three years, and she'll be the one to carry the baby. She's been inseminated four times and gotten pregnant twice. Both ended in miscarriage. Her first pregnancy came, much to her surprise, on the first attempt.

"It was literally the first time I've ever had sperm in my body," she remembered. "Suddenly, it felt real, like a whole new life—this could be it, our baby, our family." But the pregnancy stopped at eight weeks.

"The first miscarriage was devastating," she said. "Even being with a woman, my wife still doesn't understand how those hormones make you [feel]. I felt like I was losing my mind a little."

As I sat listening to her, I marveled at the fact that, five years ago, we were miscarrying at the exact same time. Working side by side, bleeding side by side, each secretly worried that, at any moment, we'd come undone. It was only months later that we found out all of this because we chose, in spite of all our hesitations, to talk about it.

My husband recently reminded me of something I'd forgotten. He said that the next day, the day after I lay on the carpet crying for an hour, when I was bleeding the heaviest, I had called him into the bathroom. I was sitting on the toilet passing large blood clots. I wiped them away and held out the piece of toilet paper to show him. I hadn't remembered doing that. I apologized because apologizing seemed like the polite thing to do, but I didn't mean it. I was glad that I had done it. That he had seen it, too.

It.

It was gelatinous, and the deepest shade of red I've ever seen—nearly black. As it fell out of me, I looked closely, both hoping and fearing that I would see something recognizable—

a tadpole, a cashew-shaped alien, a tiny eye the size of a poppy seed on something that vaguely resembled a head. I was fascinated by the stuff. It may not have been a baby, but it was part of me—something I grew with my own body. And now it was leaving me. I rolled it in my fingers. It was warm. It was not alive.

I was surprised to learn from Swanson that I was not alone in my need to touch what came out of me. In fact, touching—and being able to talk about it—is a powerful experience for many women. If a woman Swanson was interviewing had had access to the products of conception, she asked questions about it: Did you pass anything? Did you scoop it up and feel it?

"'I DID,' they'd say with huge eyes," Swanson said. "So then I'd ask them, 'What did you feel? What was the shape of it?' These are the most intimate moments I have ever experienced while counseling women. They want to tell that story, but they don't get many places to tell it."

For me, the most difficult part of that second pregnancy loss was attempting to make sense of so many new and entirely unrecognizable feelings. I found myself grieving someone I had never known, someone who, to be honest, I never even thought of as a person. How (not to mention why) do you mourn someone who never came into being?

"Women will ask themselves, 'What did I lose?'" Swanson told me. "Some will say 'not a darn thing,' others will say 'my child.' Everybody has to come to terms with what was lost and gained."

I remember my mother driving my husband and me to the

airport on Christmas morning, when we left for Little Rock. We had told her about the miscarriage the day before. Just as she was about to get back in the car, she waved and said cheerfully: "Have fun! Made in Memphis! Made in Memphis!"

I felt her love, but it didn't bring me much comfort. That came a few weeks later while talking to my friend Monica on the phone. After going through a miscarriage several months earlier, she was pregnant again.

"If I have another miscarriage, I'm done," she told me matter-of-factly.

Until then, no conversation I'd had or reading I'd done had left any room for the possibility of not trying over and over to get pregnant again. There seemed to be no space for the possibility of finding peace in a life without a baby. I realized then that if I lost more pregnancies, I wouldn't be going to any great lengths to have a child.

My former coworker, the one who has had two miscarriages, told me that she has also made peace—both with the fact that she might not be able to carry a baby, and that she and her wife are determined to meet their child. They'll keep trying, or they'll adopt, or they'll wait until her wife is ready to get pregnant. Miscarriage might stop her from having a baby, but it won't stop her from having a family.

When it comes to pregnancy loss, there is no script to follow. To help a woman navigate it, you don't need to offer advice or perspective. It is enough to show up, however awkwardly, and be there. To listen.

"What does it take to lean into it, to allow your body to go through the emotions that come from doing what we're hardwired to do?" Swanson wondered aloud at one point. "Women were made for birth and life and death," she added. "In the moment of miscarriage, birth and life and death come through us."

Getting pregnant with my daughter came as a shock, mainly because, like many other women in the months after a pregnancy loss, I was still grappling with fears that I was somehow fundamentally flawed. Was I too old? Had I waited too long? Did all those years of birth control permanently alter my uterus and hormones? Maybe my husband and I were a great romantic match but, genetically, a disastrous and doomed pair. Even though my worries were somewhat irrational, through the semi-distorted lens of loss, they made as much sense as anything else.

On a cold morning two months after my second pregnancy loss, I stood in the darkness of my bedroom on the phone with my doctor. I was the same slight mess I had been for weeks, only now I was pregnant. My first thought was if there was any greater chance that I would miscarry. I had already Googled this weeks before and knew that the risk was about 25 percent, barely higher than someone who has never lost a pregnancy, but it didn't stop me from asking.

"This probably isn't what you want to hear," my doctor said. "But I wouldn't consider you abnormal until this"— pregnancy loss—"happened to you three times in a row."

"So what do I do now?" I asked.

"Live your life. Come see me in a month."

Despite his reassurances, I spent that month—and the two months after—still suspicious that I might actually be abnormal. As much as I tried to live my life—to be grateful for and enjoy this unexpected pregnancy—I was anxious and worried that the stress might cause me to miscarry again. I waited until I was fourteen weeks pregnant with the little being that would become my daughter before I started telling people. And even then, I was still scared. I don't remember when exactly I let go of it, but I do know that, when I told others, it was their happiness that began to make the pregnancy seem viable and real. They seemed to have nothing but hope and belief. Perhaps it was that warmth that slowly melted my fear.

We are often told to accept life's difficult circumstances, in part because we can learn from them. Gradually, we think of them less as things that happened but as things that are a part of us. The same can be true for pregnancy loss.

Weeks after talking to Kristen Swanson, I couldn't stop thinking about something she said—that birth and life and death exist in women's bodies simultaneously.

I picture pregnancy loss as a primordial river rushing through me; it carries forces so big, they eclipse my imagination. It runs through my femoral artery and vena cava, through my spleen, my brain, and the chambers of my heart. At first, this force is strong like rapids, flooding everything. With time it slows, but it never goes away. It rearranges my cells like stones in a riverbed. It never stops running, even after I can no longer see or feel it.

Miscarriage helped me understand that we become mothers not, as books and websites tell us, when our babies reach the size of an avocado or butternut squash but simply when we declare ourselves so. I cannot argue with my friend who, having lost a pregnancy and given birth to two babies, considers herself, always, a mother of three. That is her life, the reality her body knows with certainty.

Someone once suggested that if I hadn't lost a pregnancy, I wouldn't have the beautiful child I have now. She was trying to make me feel better, I think, or to help me make sense of things. It was a mistake. I remember looking at her face and thinking that if I hadn't experienced that loss, I wouldn't be the person I am now.

II

TWO OF YOU

CHAPTER 5

THE BEST-LAID PLANS

Just after nine a.m. on March 6, 2013, a distant cousin of mine, Luna, went into labor. She built a comfortable nest for herself and climbed in. From 9:14 to 9:39, people around Luna heard her "intermittent high-pitched, soft vocalisations."[1] Fifty-eight minutes later, at 10:04 a.m., with her girlfriends looking on, Luna gave birth to her daughter, Leah.

Luna is a bonobo living in Salonga National Park in the Democratic Republic of the Congo. If only labor were as straightforward for the over four million people who give birth in the United States each year.

We share 98 percent of the same DNA as chimpanzees and bonobos such as Luna, which makes them our closest animal relatives. But while the labors of great apes typically last just two hours, the labor of a first-time human mother, though it varies widely, may last up to sixteen hours or more. Our births go on significantly longer than those of any other mammal, with medical procedures and hospitalization now also a routine part of the process. (Humans, like chimpanzees, also live in male-dominated societies marked by competition and aggression, sometimes lethal, between different groups. Bonobos live in matriarchal cultures that are more peaceful, egalitarian, and sexually free—and mothers typically give birth with female companions nearby.)

While we share a vast amount of genetic material with these highly intelligent and sensitive primates, our bodies differ in a few crucial ways that have profound effects on the way we give birth. Bonobos, chimps, and gorillas are big animals with roomy pelvises. Their babies are comparatively small and travel, effortlessly, out the spacious, direct path that runs from the uterus through the vagina to the outside world. A baby gorilla stays in the exact same position through birth—head down, facing its mother's stomach—and comes out looking up. In contrast, the top of the female human pelvis is the widest part—running from hip to hip—while its bottom is narrow and, to make things more complicated, widest from front to back. To make it to the outside, our babies are required to turn their heads, rotate their bodies, collapse their skull and shoulder bones, and contort themselves in a series of improbable, complex moves. It's a human obstacle course. Oh, also: their heads are considerably larger than our vaginas.

As humans parted evolutionary ways with our primate cousins over millennia, our pelvises got smaller while our heads got bigger. These are just two aspects of human anatomy, but they have outsize impacts on childbirth. For the last few decades, this evolutionary hypothesis of childbirth, called the obstetrical dilemma, has provided a framework for understanding how and why childbirth—which seems like it should unfurl as an instinctual, straightforward process—has become so complex.[2]

The last few weeks of my pregnancy felt like an eternity. I was a bulging, leaky bag of flesh. I dragged my tired, bloated body with its hemorrhoids and swollen feet and hands around each day, slowly inching toward my due date. I wanted the baby out as much as I struggled to imagine how that would happen and what my life would look like after it was all over. When my due date came and went, I began to think I might stay pregnant forever.

What I didn't know then was that due dates are bullshit. Or at least only a very rough idea of when you might give birth. According to the American Pregnancy Association, only about 5 percent of babies are actually born on their estimated due date.[3] The "estimated" part is key: A due date is based on the gestational age of a fetus, which itself is an estimation based on average fetal measurements. (And averages are just that—averages. Many numbers fall above and below.) Furthermore, gestational age is based not on the date of conception (because the actual date of conception is rarely known) but on the first day of the last known menstrual period. For people with a regular period, conception typically occurs eleven to twenty-one days after their last period began. Calculations are based on the average twenty-eight-day menstrual cycle, although cycle lengths vary widely from person to person and not everyone gets a reliable period.[4] Obviously, all of this involves a lot of estimations and approximations. It would be much more accurate, not to mention honest, for expecting mothers to be offered a four-week window during which to expect the arrival of their baby.

Due dates are appealing because they give us a target to plan around. But they can also keep us obsessively focused on a single day while our babies couldn't care less about calendars and deadlines. To better estimate due dates, we'd first need to better understand what makes labor commence.

So how do we know when the body is ready to go into labor? We don't. Even after millions of years of human reproduction, we're still not sure what makes things happen. Or when. Or why.

Newer research suggests that the onset of labor is the result of a metabolic stalemate between mother and baby, a struggle of supply and demand. At some point, the large and rapidly developing fetus maxes out the nutritional and energetic supply of its mother. Rather than starve, the baby decides to make a run for it, opting to have its needs met outside the womb. This reasoning, called the energetics of gestation and growth hypothesis, is one that scientists are now exploring further.[5] This supports increasing evidence that labor is initiated not by anything a mother does but by the fetus, which releases hormones that act upon the placenta and, in turn, the uterus.[6] Contrary to what legions of people in Internet forums suggest, eating spicy food, walking sideways up and down stairs, drinking castor oil, and shoving capsules of evening primrose oil up your vagina are unlikely to smoothly jump-start labor unless your fetus has already decided that it is ready to be born.

Increasingly, childbirth educators, books, and websites encourage expectant parents to write birth plans and spell out exactly how they want their labors and deliveries to unfold. Birth plans can include things such as preferences on pain relief, what positions you'd like to use, who will be present in the birthing room, who will catch the baby, when to initiate skin-to-skin contact, and if you want to try to breast-feed immediately. These plans can be invaluable: they help you clarify what is important to you and mitigate some of the fear of the unknown. They also provide something tangible that the people caring for you might feel obliged to follow. But committing too rigidly to a birth plan can also run directly counter to what birth itself is: utterly resistant to control.

By planning and visualizing and typing things up in a document, we hope to manifest the birth we want. Sometimes people get the birth they hope for; sometimes they do not. Trouble arises when we forget that our bodies—and our babies—have just as much influence on the circumstances of our childbirth as our minds do. I know, because this is exactly what happened to me.

I planned for a drug-free, intervention-free birth (complete with a tidy, one-page birth plan with bullet points), an admittedly cumbersome jumble of words that, no matter what, I will always prefer to the shorter, more common phrase "natural childbirth." A baby born of its mother's body is natural, whether it's pushed through her vagina or pulled out of her uterus. Cesarean sections can be lifesaving for both mother and child. For my mother, who was born with rare, congenital vaginal and uterine septa, as well as for her babies, my brothers and myself, Cesarean birth was the only viable, natural option. For the many women who have uterine fibroids and have undergone surgery to remove them, a C-section may be the safe, natural option. Labeling unmedicated vaginal birth as "natural" creates a false binary.

The C-section rate in America rose dramatically between 1996 and 2011. On its own, this fact isn't troubling, but during that time the rates of maternal and infant death did not decline. According to the American Congress of Obstetricians and Gynecologists (ACOG), this "raises significant concern that cesarean delivery is overused."[7] While it is now widely agreed that the Cesarean birth rate in the United States—33 percent in 2011—is higher than it needs to be, it remains an essential procedure for many.

Throughout our pregnancies, we receive conflicting information and mixed messages about the "right" and "wrong" ways to be and become a mother. But there is perhaps no other point that is as fraught with these contradictory, moralizing messages as labor and delivery.

On one side, mothers are portrayed as naked goddesses whose auras glow as they roam through fields of grass and squat in birthing tubs, strong and admirable. As much as these images promote the idea that giving birth like this is the purest, most normal way, all the books, classes, herbal products, aromatherapy candles, and curated Instagram accounts comprise an industry that sells this belief to women. This commerce relies on an implied shadow image of mothers who experience medicated birth lying on their backs, passive, awash in faded blue hospital garments, tied up to tubes, weak and inferior. On the other side, the medical industry benefits from the image that childbirth is inherently dangerous, emphasizing that if an emergency occurs, the baby or mother may die and *why would you even want to take that risk?* It exploits the inherent uncertainty of birth and the insecurity that accompanies having to make important, high-stakes decisions. This vision of "medicated" birth sells its patients a sense of security and superiority over others who are comparatively reckless and foolish.

We are told that giving birth is the safest and most normal human process there is. And yet, we are also told that for babies who find themselves naturally in breech positions (bottom or feet first), or with larger than average heads, or not born by forty-two weeks, vaginal delivery isn't safe, and we'll need interventions to guarantee our health.

The truth is that birth is both a normal, everyday occurrence and a significant medical event. It can be many things at once. It is, for some women, a spiritual experience that connects them with a sense of the divine. For others, the sheer feat of mental and physical fortitude offers a profound sense of bodily power and accomplishment. And for others, it is scary and psychologically devastating. Birth is also, even at its smoothest and easiest, physically traumatic.

As a culture, we have no collective definition of "safe" when it comes to bringing our children into this world. Do you feel safest in a hospital or in your home? Would you feel more secure giving birth in a rented blow-up tub in your living room or in your bed, on the sheets you sleep in every night? Or would you prefer a bed with nurses nearby, a sterile operating table? The answer is different for each of us. "Safe" can be synonymous with all of these environments.

And yet, no matter how comfortable, state-of-the-art, or "safe" the place you give birth is, there is also the shameful reality that the United States has the highest maternal death rate of any developed country in the world. I'm not trying to scare you unnecessarily. While death in pregnancy and child-birth is rare here, it is nowhere close to rare enough. Every year between seven hundred and nine hundred women die in childbirth, while almost sixty-five thousand nearly die.[8]

"In every other wealthy country, and many less affluent ones, maternal mortality rates have been falling," a 2017 *ProPublica* investigation found. "But in the U.S., maternal deaths increased from 2000 to 2014."[9]

Even more alarming is the racial disparity within these deaths: Black mothers are three to four times more likely to die from pregnancy-related causes than white mothers.[10] And overall, nonwhite women are far more likely to experience complications and a range of less favorable obstetrical out-comes.[11] It's a reality many of us have to contend with at some point: that what happens to us at the end of pregnancy and childbirth may look different because we look different from the average white woman. It's an extra layer of consideration and stress that goes into where and how we decide to give birth.

The choices we make—ob-gyn, midwife, family doctor, home birth, birthing center, hospital—don't reflect our strength of character, inherent goodness, or health. They are personal choices that often reflect the culture we come from, what we can afford, what provider we happen to feel most comfortable with. Instead of approaching these choices as being better or worse than others, we should be doing our best to make sure they are all as accessible, comfortable, and safe as possible.

Childbirth is beautiful, but it is not pretty. It is grisly and life affirming, glorious and deadly. It requires you to open, to rip apart both physically and emotionally, and allows the scent of death to seep through those tears and fissures. Whatever form it takes, however long it takes, it is also the means to an ecstatic end.

While American culture doesn't like to acknowledge this undeniable link between life and death, it's certainly not a new idea. Orthodox Jews recite the same prayer of thanksgiving—*benching gomel*—after childbirth that they do after surviving a near-death experience. The Hindu goddess Durga is revered as the divine mother of the universe; she holds the power both to create and to destroy life. Ancient Egyptians worshipped Taweret, a goddess whose body combined the soft features of a fertile woman with those of the fierce crocodile and hippopotamus. Taweret protected women during childbirth; her image was carved into the instruments, including wands made of hippopotamus ivory, that Egyptian midwives used during childbirth. And throughout history, midwives—those who guided new life into the world—were often the same women who tended to the people and bodies on their way out.

I went into birth uncertain but unafraid. I didn't know what would happen, but I felt prepared, confident that I could birth my child how I wanted. I discovered my body and my daughter had other plans, ones that took me to a dark place where fear and danger took on another dimension. I ended up grateful for the interventions I had not wanted. I didn't necessarily want to learn all of this, but I didn't have a choice.

*

Five days after my due date, my labor began at around eight p.m. As I was sitting on the couch watching *Monday Night Football*, I started feeling mild cramps. Knowing labor could be a long haul, I went to bed to try to rest. I barely slept, the cramping happening every ten minutes, increasing in intensity. They weren't terrible, thirty or so seconds of fierce tightening that I could still breathe easily through until they passed. They went on all night, until the sun came up, when suddenly they disappeared.

In the morning I told my husband, who had slept through all of it. Was this labor? This had to be labor, right? If so, why was it stopping? We called the birthing center at the hospital where we were going to deliver, and a nurse told us to come in so we could find out what was going on.

At the hospital, we sat in a cramped space between flimsy curtains for over an hour. I wasn't having any contractions and started to regret being there. Finally, two residents came in to check me. They didn't ask many questions—the particulars of what brought me there weren't that important, I learned, only what was happening in that moment.

"I can't even feel your cervix," a resident with a thick black beard told me after shoving his gloved fingers up my vagina. "You're not in labor. There's no way you're having this baby today. You can go home."

I cried on the drive back, feeling disappointed and embarrassed, wondering if the residents were now laughing me off as some sort of hysterical first-time mom. My husband looked at me and said simply, "You've never done this before. How are you supposed to know?"

That night, starting at nine o'clock, the contractions came again, ten minutes apart, each one feeling stronger than the last. This night was different. With each contraction, I put both my hands against the wall and bent over, breathing slowly and, when that wasn't enough, braying softly like a donkey. I was surprised by the sound, one that I'd never heard myself make before. I fell into a heap on the bed after each one, half-asleep, until I was stirred to action again. I got up and went to the wall and repeated the whole process. Hours passed, filled with nothing more than getting up, bending over, braying, and lying back down. Having thoughts seemed irrelevant; I just followed the actions my body told me to take.

By sunrise, the contractions had stopped again. It was Wednesday morning, and I was officially forty-one weeks pregnant.

That morning I went to my appointment with our family doctor, who would be delivering the baby. I remember having scheduled the appointment weeks before, thinking that I wouldn't need it because my baby, born on or before its due date, would already be here. My doctor examined me and told me my cervix was three centimeters dilated.

I was relieved. I hadn't endured all those contractions for nothing! Things were progressing, albeit slowly, but my body was at least handling its business. I'd be in labor soon. On the way home, I felt hopeful. I reminded myself to trust my body, to trust birth, as I had surely read in *Spiritual Midwifery* or some other Ina May Gaskin book.

Only weeks later, after I gave birth, after a few hours of sleep-deprived Googling, did I discover that there was a name for what I was going through: prodromal labor. Prodromal labor is something like purgatory—definitely closer to hell than heaven, though. It is occasionally called false labor, but it is, in fact, labor, one that happens before you go into the full-blown, active stage. It occurs often when babies, rather than being head down and facing the mother's back (the ideal position), are in breech or posterior (head down, facing the mother's abdomen) positions. This suggests that the contractions of prodromal labor—regular, but not enough to fully dilate the cervix or push the baby down the birth canal—are the body's way of trying to maneuver the baby into a more favorable place.

Before birth, the question at the top of nearly every first-time mother's list of questions is, "What will the contractions feel like?" The pain of contractions was probably what terrified and fascinated me most about birth. And yet, for all my wondering, it was impossible to understand the sensations until I was experiencing them. Looking back, I wish I had spent more time trying to understand the purpose—and power—of my uterus and its contractions.

The uterus—a uniquely female organ—not only shelters

the fetus but grows along with it. A normal, healthy uterus is small—about three inches long and two inches wide—but it expands exponentially throughout pregnancy. To use the fruit-size comparisons favored by most online pregnancy resources, the uterus grows from roughly the size of an orange that sits deep within the pelvis to a watermelon that will displace organs such as the stomach and lungs, eventually grazing the rib cage. It's not just the size of the uterus that is significant but also its volume. A pregnant uterus expands to over forty-five times its usual capacity: the volume of a healthy uterus is typically under 100 milliliters (ml), but by twenty weeks of pregnancy it reaches 1,000 ml and, at forty weeks, a whopping 4,500 ml.[12]

The lining of the uterus, the endometrium, is a mucous membrane lined with blood vessels where the embryo attaches and the placenta grows. It is surrounded by a layer of smooth muscle, the myometrium, which transforms from a stable, relatively static entity into the tireless, forceful workhorse of labor. Uterine contractions, like blood pressure, are measured in millimeters of mercury (mm Hg) called Montevideo units. At 80 mm Hg, when contractions are considered "strong," the pressure is equal to 1.5 pounds per square inch on the baby's head. Contractions can reach up to 110 mm Hg, or 2.12 pounds per square inch—sometimes even higher.

That level of force accomplishes a few things: pushing a baby's head and body downward toward the vagina, thinning and opening the cervix, and, astonishingly, transfusing the fetus with its own blood.

A full-term placenta holds about six ounces of a fetus's

blood, which is about half of a newborn's blood volume. The infant needs that blood to be in its body when it makes its way to the outside. So how does it get into the baby's body in time for it to be born? The mighty uterus and its contractions, which squeeze the placenta, force blood through the umbilical vein and into the fetus. As the uterus steadily increases the pressure it places on the placenta, the organ continues to shrink, and the amount of blood inside the fetus grows until it has what it needs to take its first breath and utter its first cry outside its mother's body.[13] The contractions we must endure—for hours, sometimes days—do so much more than cause pain.

On the third night of my prodromal labor, I readied myself for the next battle and, sure enough, at nine p.m., the contractions started again, five minutes or so apart. I was exhausted, and these contractions felt much harder to manage than the previous night's. After every contraction, I felt the urge to pee, so I would sit on the toilet as a little urine trickled out of me each time. I didn't think anything of it. I knew people often involuntarily pooped while in labor, so I figured they must pee a lot, too.

Around four thirty a.m., I got up from bed and walked to the bathroom to pee. Just as I was turning on the light, I suddenly felt nauseous and rushed to the toilet to throw up. As I vomited, a gush of warm liquid came out of my vagina, rushing down my thighs and splashing onto the bath mat. I promptly threw up again, grinning as I bent over the toilet bowl. I was overjoyed. Finally, I remember thinking, now things can really get going.

"My water just broke!" I yelled.

When we arrived at the hospital a few hours later, a test was administered to confirm that the liquid that came out of me was amniotic fluid. Minutes later, a nurse ducked behind the curtains to tell me that it was not, in fact, amniotic fluid that had come out of me.

"Oh no, it was amniotic fluid," I told her. Who was this woman?

I am trusting my body, I wanted to scream at her. *My body will not be fucking with me today. And neither will you.*

"What else could it be?"

An ultrasound machine was wheeled in so they could check my amniotic fluid level. Before she began, the nurse instructed me to go to the bathroom and "empty my bladder." I went in, peed my little trickle, and came back.

As I lay back on the hospital bed, the nurse passed the ultrasound wand over my lower abdomen. Suddenly she stopped and said, "When I asked you to empty your bladder, that meant to urinate. Did you understand that?" I'm sure she was asking nicely, but all I heard was condescension.

"Yes, I understood you," I said. "I peed."

"Are you sure?" she asked.

"Yes, I'm sure," I snapped.

Something was clearly wrong.

"Look at the image on the screen," the nurse told me, pointing. "This is your bladder—and it is full of liquid."

Another nurse was called in and they told me that the baby was likely obstructing my bladder. As for my "water breaking," well, that had actually been urine that, trapped inside me, could only be expelled by the force of my vomiting.

The only way to know for sure what was happening was to catheterize me. I consented, and they drained what felt like a small lake of urine. I saw it fill up the pan, and I felt relieved.

After it was done, I asked if I could go home. A resident looked at me and laughed.

"No. Just because we drained your bladder, it doesn't mean the problem is solved," he said. "Your baby is still obstructing it."

Like everyone, I have a more complicated relationship with my body than I would like. I am grateful to it, often admire it, but I don't always like it. I sometimes think, in sickness or injury, that it has failed me, even as it is working quietly, steadfastly to heal itself.

Pregnancy—and preparing for labor and childbirth—put me in a certain awe of my body. It was a tired body, yes, but also one that literally pulsed and bulged with life: fetal kicks, hiccups, turns, and rolls. But there was always the nagging question of whom, ultimately, it was working for. A pregnant mother and her fetus are connected, yes, but they are also looking out for their own needs. Suddenly, at forty-one weeks, I found myself wondering if my body would throw me under the bus for the sake of my baby. Would it have to choose, and, if so, could I trick it to side with me?

My baby, in its attempts to get out of my body, was wreaking havoc on it, literally getting in the way of my being able to perform the most basic of functions. If it wouldn't let me pee in peace, what wouldn't it block, crawl, drag, and pull with it on its way out?

We waited for our doctor to show up. He explained that he

couldn't just send me home. I was well past my due date and couldn't urinate unassisted. That was an issue. If I wanted to go home, it would have to be with a catheter and a bag of urine hanging out of me. He suggested that I be admitted and that we start an induction.

I looked at my husband in tears. I couldn't face the thought of checking in right then and there, of obliterating the birth I had planned from its onset. So I invoked a proud tradition of my ancestors. Like the many Filipina women in my family who came before me, I bargained. But instead of the price of a kilo of mangoes or a purse from a market vendor, I haggled for the best deal I could get for my autonomy.

What if, I proposed to my doctor, we went home for a few hours? No catheter. I could get my things in order, go for a walk, give this baby one last chance to start this birth on its own. If not, we'd come back that night for the induction. He agreed.

As soon as we walked out of the hospital doors, I felt momentarily free. We walked a few of the blocks around the hospital, past our old apartment building, the Trader Joe's we used to shop at. It seemed strange that anyone would be buying groceries, running ordinary errands. I realized then that I was already in another universe; I was just visiting this one for a few minutes.

We got in our car and drove home, where I walked in the door and stuck a finger down my throat as I sat on the toilet, making myself gag so I could pee.

I packed my hospital bag: the tiny brown onesie, maroon pants, and green fleece booties that I had picked out for our baby's going-home outfit. Something cute and gender neutral because we didn't know what we were having. I texted my doula, Sage, and arranged for her to meet us at the hospital later. Then I drew a hot bath and sent my closest girlfriends a long text explaining what was about to happen. "See you on the other side," I typed with my thumbs, sending the words out in a blue bubble to land on their screens.

Then I crawled into the tub, closed my eyes, and floated— away from everything and everyone, somewhere deep into myself, where, although the next twenty-four hours would bring me into close contact with dozens of nurses and doctors, I remained alone.

*

In my birth plan, I had requested that no IV port be placed when I checked in, which was the hospital's policy. My doctor, somewhat reluctantly, made a note in my chart. After checking into the hospital and getting settled in our room, I was given Pitocin, the synthetic form of the natural hormone oxytocin that is used to help initiate labor. It was administered through the freshly placed intravenous needle in my wrist. My labor began with the very thing I had fought against.

I was familiar with the statistics: women who are induced have higher rates of interventions such as epidurals and C-sections. I feared that once I agreed to an induction, I'd end up with every possible intervention that I didn't want. Tubes and ports and needles and drips, not just me and my body, but my body piped and tethered to machines.

My body responded well to the Pitocin. Within an hour, I was experiencing powerful contractions, coming close together. I was ready for them. I found my rhythm. I was no longer surprised by the low-toned moans I was making; it was my own private language. I still couldn't pee without gagging myself, but for the first few hours I managed to resist having a catheter put in so I could labor in a tub.

I know my husband and my doula were right there with me, talking to me, pouring cups of water on my back as I labored. I know because there are pictures to prove it. But I really don't remember it. He tells me that I "wasn't there." I was in my body, but in a completely new way. I had the feeling of being in some dark place low down. My baby was there, too, but it was nowhere within my reach. As for my brain—my consciousness—it was also somewhere else entirely, but I saw no use in trying to locate it.

After about two hours, I had progressed to five centimeters. I felt so good—strong, accomplished. I was sure that I would be fully dilated soon, that I'd be able to push this baby out just as I had planned. But another two hours later—after contractions that were coming back-to-back, two at a time with only a minute or so to rest in between each set, I was still at five centimeters. Around two or three in the morning, a resident came by with the unfortunate job of telling me that she thought I should get an epidural. I looked at her, didn't say a word, turned away, and never looked at her again.

Thoughts went through me, though I didn't have the ability to say them out loud: *I don't know how long I can do this*

*for. But isn't that the point? What if I have another hour, an-
other day in me? I want to find out.*

Later, my doctor appeared in the room, but I was too busy
riding wave after wave of contractions, bellowing as I held
on to my husband, to speak to him. I remember turning to
him a few times, thinking I'd get some words out, but I never
managed. More thoughts flowed through me.

*How does time pass? What is time even for? Does time really
exist? These are just moments that distend, like my body, past a
point of recognition, into something else entirely.*

When I finally had more than a minute between contractions to focus on my doctor's face, we talked. He had been in
the room for almost two hours. He told me that I was doing
great, that he'd been watching. But I was still only at five
centimeters. He suggested the epidural and told me gently
that the only way I was going to have a chance at the vaginal
delivery I wanted was if I got the medication and rested.

"You can rest, and then after you have rested, you can
push," he said.

I consented. At around six in the morning, an anesthesiologist came in to administer the epidural. I barely remember the process by which she threaded the thin tube, a spinal
catheter, between my vertebrae. I only remember feeling very
cold and being surprised as I receded further into myself, into
a tiny hole, perhaps as small as the one poked into my spine.

I lay down, exhausted, unable to feel much, and slept
for hours. My support team slept, too. When I woke up, a
third set of nurses was by my side. They started me on Pitocin again, and the contractions came again—strong, they

told me, based on the readout of my new uterine catheter. I couldn't feel them.

After several hours—three, four, who knows?—they checked me. Six centimeters. Progress, but not much. After another three hours, another check. Still six.

In the early evening, things started happening. Just not the sorts of things you want to happen. I developed a fever and my white blood cell count rose. There was an infection brewing in my bladder, which was still being drained by a catheter.

My doctor told me that he was going to hold off on diagnosing the infection for a bit. He also told me that if the fever and infection progressed, my labor would be considered high-risk. I'd have to have surgery, and the baby would not be allowed to come back to the room with me after delivery. It would be sent to the nursery.

Delivery. I had forgotten about that part, that it was the goal, that it was even a possibility.

When my doctor said that it was "getting close to the time that you might want to start thinking about other options," I knew what he meant. I also knew that he would give me time to come to a decision. I asked for a few minutes of privacy and, when the room was empty, I told my husband, "Let's get the C-section."

He looked at me, his eyes filling with tears, and said, "Are you sure? I know how much you wanted to have the vaginal birth. I know you can do it."

He was doing exactly what I had asked him to do. To remind me of what I wanted, to be held accountable to myself. It broke me a little to hear him say it. What he didn't know, and what I had unconsciously come to realize, was that I was already a different person. I hadn't delivered the baby yet, wasn't officially a mother yet, but labor had already changed me.

Why had I wanted a vaginal birth so badly in the first place? Because, above all, I believed in what my body was built to do. I wanted to witness—to experience—just what it was capable of.

But there were other reasons, too. Because I had taken a birthing class that strongly reinforced my beliefs. Because my best friends had done it. And because, being a sort of nerd about biology and bodily gore, I had gotten really into learning about the human—and vaginal—microbiome. Your microbiome is made up of the trillions of bacteria that populate nearly every part of your body and that are unique to just you.

There are more microbes in your intestinal tract than there are stars in the galaxy. Microbes far outnumber our own cells, and they populate all the parts of us that play a pivotal role in reproduction. The origins of the placenta can be traced back to a virus. Microbes predate human life by literally billions of years and have been evolving right along with us since we showed up on earth.

In the late nineteenth century, after the spread of several diseases was linked to certain bacteria and germs, microbes were recast as symbols of illness, uncleanliness, and death. That bad reputation persists today, even though dangerous pathogens make up a minuscule fraction of microbial life. While as a society we're still pretty germophobic, in pregnancy and motherhood we are beginning to see a shift in understanding.

During vaginal birth, a baby's journey down the birth canal serves as its intimate introduction to its mother's vaginal microbiome, the distinct combination of bacteria that go on to help the growing human deal with infection, train its immune system, and help it process food.

"Very flexible, rather like a glove, the vagina covers the newborn's every surface, hugging its soft skin as it passes through. And with that hugging a transfer occurs," Dr. Martin Blaser writes rather poetically in his book *Missing Microbes*. "The baby's skin is a sponge, taking up the vaginal microbes rubbing against it. . . . The first fluids the baby sucks in contain mom's microbes, including some fecal matter. Labor is not an antiseptic process."[14]

After vaginal birth, an infant's microbiome closely resembles that of the mother's vagina. For years, the lactobacillus species of bacteria was believed to dominate the vaginal microbiomes of most women. But newer research has found tremendous variety among the vaginal microbiomes across ethnicities. Research also suggests that babies born via C-section, who are more likely to experience health issues including asthma and allergies, might be at greater risk because they lack the same bacterial exposure as their vaginally born counterparts.[15]

I loved the idea that the gunk of my vagina, which as a child I had been taught was dirty and had always felt self-conscious about, could be critical to a baby's health. (Perhaps if I had known it was a possibility, I would have requested, like other mothers, to have my vagina swabbed and then rubbed on my baby's face so she could have gotten that first dose of microbes.)

But, as much as all of that sounded great, four days into the throes of labor, I let go of all of it. The bacteria in my bladder took priority over the ones in my vagina. The only things I really needed were to survive and hold my baby.

Within minutes of making my decision, I was being wheeled into the operating room. I couldn't feel anything. Yet my senses were working overtime—the sounds of rubber gloves and metal tools, the fuzzy antiseptic smell and taste of nothing but dryness in my mouth, and the too-bright lights nearly canceling each other out. I heard my baby before I saw her. She was screaming, it seemed, from inside me. At least four other people put their hands on her before I did, which felt wrong, but nothing about this situation felt quite right.

When things go well, it is easy to celebrate our bodies. But when things go poorly, or not how we imagined, it becomes much harder. I could look back and think about the ways my body disappointed me—and I did, a few times. But whenever I went down that road, I found that it was a dead-end street that made me feel terrible. Hating my body remains a waste of time. At some point, just for the purpose of survival, I chose, deliberately, to focus on all the things my body did right, what it did so well on my behalf. Everything it tried to do.

My body had prepared itself for vaginal birth, releasing relaxin (the most perfectly named substance in the world) to loosen the ligaments of my pubic bones so my pelvis would give way during delivery. Relaxin isn't so sophisticated that it can target specific bones, and instead it acts upon the whole body. Throughout pregnancy, my hands and wrists widened and filled with fluid, pressing on nerves that made my fingers tingle. I waited tables with numb hands for months. My feet grew a half size and never returned to their previous state. I am reminded of the work my body did almost every morning when I reach past a beloved pair of brown leather boots on the shoe rack that I'll never be able to wear again but still cannot bear to throw away.

I think of my cervix, which for more than twenty-five years has shape-shifted week after week, month after month, with my cycle—softening and hardening, sitting high or low, opening and closing. Made of collagen, at the start of pregnancy it ramped up its production and packed its proteins tightly together. It bulked up, became stronger, and then lodged itself firmly in place to protect what was growing inside me. As my pregnancy came to a close, it produced an enzyme to kill off the collagen and smooth muscle that gave it its strength. It became porous and filled itself with water, making it softer—riper—so that it would be able to open up for my baby to pass through. It never fully dilated, but it did make it two-thirds of the way there, and that's not nothing. Soon after birth, it began rebuilding, accumulating collagen again, taking up its post as a gatekeeper to my most vulnerable, powerful place.

When things go badly, isn't that the time to be even more understanding and generous with our bodies, with ourselves? Isn't that the most critical time to try to understand and appreciate all that our bodies do for us and, if we can't do that, to accept things and move forward? Acceptance doesn't happen overnight, maybe ever, but for me, the process of trying is essential.

*

Just before they began sewing me closed, the anesthesiologist, a professorial older white man I'd never met before but who I suddenly trusted with my life, leaned in and told me, "You're going to feel a tremendous amount of pressure now. Some women say it is like an elephant stepping on their stomach. I can give you something if you need it."

And then, suddenly, there it was. The pressure. The bearing down. The suffocating, dull, unrelenting pushing—not just on my stomach, but also on my chest, my heart, my ability to think, possibly to continue living. I started breathing frantically and I looked at him with panicked eyes. "I'm going to need that now."

Afterward, back in our room, our doctor told us that our daughter had been in a posterior position, which may have been why she got stuck. He also told me, having seen the insides of my body, that my bladder had been obstructed in two different places. It distended upward significantly and, at the time of surgery, the top section still held days-old urine that the catheters could never have reached.

"I've actually never seen anything like it," he remarked.

To this day, I have no idea why my baby got stuck, if in those nights of trying to wiggle her way into a better position, it was she who blocked my bladder, or my bladder that got in her way. Or if they just found themselves in some awkward, inextricable embrace. My doctor, who has delivered many babies over several decades, queried his colleagues, but no one could come up with any explanation for why it happened, why I needed every intervention that I did not want. Had she stubbornly refused to turn her head, or did my own body— the only protection she had ever known—stand in her way?

Looking back, I realize that I no longer care. It is just our story.

Back in the operating room, when my husband laid our daughter on my chest, it only took her a minute, in spite of her scrunched eyes and incessant high-pitched squawking, to scoot herself over to my breast. I felt so grateful to her for that. For pulling and drawing me out of myself at last.

For knowing I was her mother, that it had been me—her, us—all along.

CHAPTER 6

TAKE CARE

Back in my hospital room after surgery, I stared at my daughter as she nursed. I felt high, as though I was on drugs. (I was.) I was sweating profusely. A vital part of me now lived outside my body. I looked at it in disbelief, the glow of the red neon Safeway sign across the street seeping in through the windows, pulsing gently at the edges of my peripheral vision.

The nurse on shift, whose name I can no longer remember, disrupted the spell. She came on just before I decided to have the C-section and we never had a chance to establish a real rapport. We were intimately acquainted, however, as she was the person who shaved off my pubic hair just before I was wheeled into surgery.

"I saw your birth plan," she said wryly, raising her eyebrows as she placed a pillow under my arm for support. "Sorry about that."

Then she leaned in closer and added, gently, "I've seen a lot of births, and *this*"—she gestured to the creature grunting and sucking on me ravenously, as it had been doing nonstop since the operating room——"doesn't happen all the time."

She turned to walk away, then paused. "One day, you might even look back and think you got a good deal."

My immediate reaction is forever lost to my drug-induced haze, but I have thought of this woman many times since. I wish I could remember her name. I wish that I could go back and thank her. I didn't realize it at the time, but she had told me, in just a few words, exactly what I needed to hear. She acknowledged the disappointment I might feel about birth and pointed out, without platitudes, the beauty that came from it. And she let me know, subtly, that my birth experience was entirely my own——no need to compare it to anyone else's.

My idealized dream of labor and delivery—and the gruesome cascade of interventions that ended up being my reality—were complete opposites. In the emotional, hormone-soaked aftermath, swimming through the nonstop deluge of *feeeeeeeeeeeelings*—overwhelming love, debilitating weakness, dumbfounded awe, bumbling incompetence—I was surprised to find that I wasn't upset about my birth. I didn't feel guilty or traumatized, as so many other women felt who also did not have the births they'd envisioned.

The question I kept coming back to was, "Why?"

It's not that I haven't struggled with it. If anything, I felt that maybe I "missed out" on something by not having a vaginal birth. Some elusive, key element of womanhood. I am certainly not missing out on any of the results of my labor—an increasingly willful child and the nonstop job of parenting. I've expelled enough blood and fluid from my vagina to last a lifetime. And yet, when I hear or read the proud stories of women who had satisfying vaginal births, I sometimes feel a sting of sadness. Occasionally I wonder if my existence as a woman is somehow incomplete. As though growing a life and giving birth were not enough.

Aside from a baby's exit from the body, there is no single experience that makes a birth "complete" or "normal" or "right." Medical interventions—inductions, C-sections, vacuum extractions—grew from the desire and necessity to preserve the health and lives of mothers and their babies. One hundred years ago, a "natural" childbirth could very well have meant injury, sickness, or death for me or my baby—or both of us.

We've allowed our understanding of childbirth to be divided into two highly polarized categories: "natural" and "medicated." We are aggressively encouraged—by our peers and childbirth educators—to believe that birth without medical intervention or pain relief is a better, more authentic, more "natural" experience of childbirth. An equally vocal set of experts is waiting to tell us to forget all of that and "just get the epidural" because childbirth is inherently painful and dangerous and, if the technology exists and is safe, why wouldn't you want to be as comfortable as possible?

The truth is that birth doesn't fall easily into one of two types. Childbirth is not a zero-sum game. It is a spectrum, with most people's experiences falling somewhere in between two extremes.

There are an infinite number of ways that childbirth can go. We feel contractions. Sometimes we endure them for longer than we ever imagined we could. Or we may find that, in its painful, merciless throes, we want relief and the opportunity to continue feeling more comfortable and rested. Maybe we are thrilled to find that the pain, while undeniable, is instructive, pointing us to a place of focus and strength we didn't know we had. We might find comfort in giving birth at home, surrounded by family, or in a setting free from any familial baggage or expectations. We may realize that we need medical assistance—and that we are fortunate to have access to it. It's the rare exception to land squarely in the "natural" or "medical" end; it's the norm to find yourself somewhere in the vast middle ground.

Who sets the standards of what "normal" or "natural" are, if these things even exist? Who decides what makes a person a woman, anyway? There is no fundamental, defining experience of womanhood. For hundreds of years, black women in the United States weren't legally considered "women," only property. There are millions of women who are physically unable to give birth or are entirely uninterested in going through the process. They are no less women than mothers.

In this day and age, you also don't need to identify as a woman to give birth. There are certainly some biological requirements, but those are simply female body parts. As of 2016, 1.4 million adults in the United States identified as transgender, double the number from the widely accepted previous estimate from 2011.[1] While no official data has been collected, a growing number of gender nonbinary people and trans men get pregnant and give birth every year.[2]

"Humans are built to have babies, so every type of human

has babies," said Simon Ellis, a Seattle-based certified nurse midwife and the coauthor of one of the only research papers to date about trans and gender variant people who have given birth. "I always knew in my heart that trans people had to have babies, because people have babies."

When we buy into the false binary of childbirth, just as when we buy into the false binary of gender, people will always fall through the gap. The idea that birth can only go one way or the other, and that bad things will happen if birth does not unfold as we think it should, does not set people up for success. Instead, they will feel that they failed—and they will feel terrible.

Of the nearly four million women who give birth each year in America, between 20 and 30 percent describe their births as traumatic.[3] They all believed, at some point during one of the most significant events of their lives, that their lives or their baby's lives were in danger, or that their physical and emotional well-being was at risk.

What if we could see birth on a spectrum that provides us the opportunity to include—and support—everyone?

Native American tribes recognized as many as five different genders across their indigenous languages. Today, Native people use the term "two spirit" to describe these gender-diverse people. Traditionally, a two-spirit person's ability to see and understand the world from multiple perspectives was believed to be a powerful gift.

Being open to the benefits of all experiences of childbirth allows us to empathize and see the perspectives of more people and to support mothers in whatever mode of birth they choose or end up having. What if we reconsider the way we think about childbirth and make our primary objective ensuring the comfort and safety of the laboring mother?

When my friend Sam told me her birth story—a full three and a half years after her daughter came into the world—she was still raw. She shook with emotion. "It was," she said, "the most traumatic thing that has ever happened to me by a long shot."

Sam hoped to have an intervention-free birth, in part because both her mother and her older sister had done so with each of their four children. She and her husband chose a midwifery practice in New York City that catered to families looking for this type of birth experience.

Sam went into labor early in the morning and labored at home for the better part of a day. Her contractions intensified steadily and started to feel acutely painful, but, after more than twelve hours, they weren't quite hitting the 4–1–1 pattern (four minutes apart, each lasting one minute, for one hour) that her midwives told her was necessary to head to the hospital. Over multiple phone calls, as she tried to explain how the pain in her back just didn't feel right, her midwife told her that if she was able to talk through her contractions at all, she wasn't ready to be admitted.

Finally, that night, exhausted and in anguish, Sam decided to trust her gut and went to the hospital. She called her midwife, who agreed to meet her there. In triage, Sam immediately requested an epidural—she was over the discomfort. She was told that there were no open beds in any rooms, so until one was available, she and her husband were left in a hallway, where they stayed, mostly unattended, for several hours. Her midwife showed up, seemed displeased by her intention to get the epidural, and then disappeared.

"I don't know where she went," Sam told me. "But I do know that, as I was laboring and just trying to get through my contractions in this hallway, people came by to tell me that I needed to be quiet."

At one point, a gush of fluid, blood, and discharge fell out of her vagina and onto the floor. No one was around, so her husband left her to find a bathroom and paper towels to wipe it up.

Eventually, Sam was moved to a room where she got her epidural, which allowed her to relax and rest. Within four hours, she went from two centimeters to fully dilated and was able to push her baby out. Her daughter came out with a bruised forehead and two black eyes ("She literally looked like a boxer"); she had been in a posterior position, which is what caused the severe back pain. During birth, Sam experienced a third-degree vaginal tear, which her midwife repaired with stitches before leaving. Soon after, a nurse came by and told her that the stitches were not done properly; they would need to be taken out and resewn. Sam was never contacted about a six-week postpartum visit.

"I went through the looking glass that day," she said. "To a harder world, not a welcoming place. I had an awakening: I cannot trust medical professionals."

As my friend told me her story, I was stunned. And then I was furious. How could this have possibly happened? Why didn't anyone just help her? That such an important, transformative event was so harrowing for her—and for so many other women—is shameful.

"It wasn't that I had interventions, or didn't have a certain kind of birth that upsets me," she said. "It was that no one was really there for me."

*

"It's not how you give birth, it's how you're cared for that really matters," Penny Simkin told me. Simkin is an internationally renowned, Seattle-based childbirth and labor support educator who has been working in the field since 1968. Over the last five decades, she estimates that she has assisted hundreds of laboring mothers as a doula and has prepared over fourteen thousand women and families for birth.

When I was pregnant, my husband and I took Simkin's eight-week-long childbirth class. It was designed for families who, while they planned to give birth in a hospital setting, were interested in low-intervention births. As I expected, the majority of our classes focused on nonmedicated comfort measures—movement, breathing, massage—that mothers and partners could use to get through the pain of labor and delivery. Over the weeks, we practiced holding on to each other as we stood and swayed like slow-dancing middle schoolers, staring into each other's eyes and counting breaths, as well as getting down on our hands and knees and rocking our hips back and forth. The curriculum also included different laboring positions and movements that women who received epidurals could use to increase their comfort and remain active, which helps a baby down the birth canal during labor.

Simkin, who lectures and offers trainings at childbirth conferences and workshops around the world, has championed the concept of labor support and brought it into mainstream consciousness. She cofounded the Doula Organization of North America, now called DONA International, as well as the professional collective for the Prevention and Treatment of Traumatic Childbirth (PATTCh).

In the early 1980s, after fifteen years of working in labor and childbirth, Simkin, a physical therapist by training, was considering a career shift. Before doing so, though, she wanted to know if her work supporting women in labor had a lasting impact on these mothers, or if they forgot the details of their births over the years. She had no formal research experience but, inspired by a research paper written by a nurse at the University of Washington on women's experiences with miscarriage, she decided to conduct her own study. She invited twenty women whom she had assisted early in her career—and whose handwritten birth stories she still had—to recount their births after many years.

"I compared the stories, and they were so consistent. I was astounded," said Simkin. "Women don't forget."

Along with telling their stories, Simkin asked the mothers to rate, on a scale of 1 to 10, how satisfied they felt with their births. A proponent of unmedicated childbirth, she expected the mothers who had, in her words, "easy, natural births" to be more satisfied than those who had "tougher, longer" labors with medical interventions.

"But it didn't work out that way," she said. "Some of the people that had easy, fast labors were very unhappy. Others had long, painful labors, and yet they felt really good about it."

Not only were some of the women with difficult births content, they also had fond, vivid memories. One woman who had severe back pain throughout her entire labor spoke at length about the nurse who stayed on after her shift was done to be there for the delivery and how, after she gave birth, the same nurse gave her a back rub. More than fifteen years later, the mother described the details of looking out the window—the sun, the clouds, the way objects moved through the sky—as the nurse tended to her.

Simkin realized then that it was not the physical act of birth itself that held the most potent memories for women, but the way they were cared for before, during, and after birth.

Her story reminded me of something I'd learned from Dr. Kristen Swanson, the professor of nursing I'd interviewed about her research on pregnancy loss. Based on interviews conducted in the early 1980s, she developed an empathy-based theory of nursing care for patients who had experienced miscarriage. When I mentioned Swanson's name to Simkin, her face lit up immediately.

"Yes, I know that name!" she said. "She's the one who wrote the paper I read. It was called *The Unborn One.*"

Penny Simkin and Kristen Swanson both live in Seattle. While they have never met, their work has affected the lives of many women on their journey through pregnancy, loss, and motherhood—including myself.

When Swanson set out to research women's experiences

with miscarriage three decades ago, she found there was no existing tool to effectively evaluate them. So she created her own. She interviewed women in an intimate setting, one-on-one, asking them all the same standard questions and allowing them time to describe the complexity of their individual feelings and experiences. Her findings drove her to pursue a nursing career dedicated to improving the care of the many women for whom pregnancy has also been marked by loss.

Simkin, too, set out, first and foremost, to listen to women's stories. In turn, her discoveries led her to devote the remainder of her career to caring for women during childbirth. She cofounded DONA with the goal of creating formal guidelines and standards for labor support.

Labor and loss are two of life's most essential processes, but that universality also holds an infinite number of individual stories and details. Swanson and Simkin created and held space for women to share these diverse experiences. What is most remarkable is that it all began with Swanson's disarmingly simple questions, questions that require us to make the time to listen to people in their own words: *What is it like? What made you feel cared for?*

What their work and research have clearly shown is that care is integral. It is a quietly radical act that dramatically affects both the obstetrical and the psychological outcomes of birth. Continuous, nonjudgmental labor support and care leads to better outcomes including lower C-section rates, less use of pain medications (which, while helpful, have their own side effects), as well as fewer vacuum- and forceps-assisted births. Labors also tend not to last as long, forty minutes shorter on average, which, when every minute-long contraction feels like an eternity, is significant.[4]

One way we might better care for women is to offer all laboring and postpartum mothers access to a doula.

The term "doula," derived from an antiquated Greek word meaning "female servant," is someone who provides support—physical, emotional, informational—for laboring mothers. Unlike nurses and midwives, doulas do not perform medical or clinical tasks. They are there only to support the mother in whatever she decides to do and to comfort her and reinforce her trust in herself.

Before Simkin and her colleagues established DONA, being a doula wasn't considered a formal profession and the scope of the work wasn't well defined. Today, doula certification and training programs are used internationally. Doulas don't need to obtain a license to practice, but most become certified through organizations such as DONA International. The number of doulas who complete DONA training each year has grown exponentially since its founding, from 750 doulas in 1994 to more than 12,000 in 2016.

Along with providing comfort measures such as touch and sustenance, doulas advocate for the client's wishes. They might encourage their clients to ask questions of health providers, to express their preferences and concerns. What doulas do not—or at least should not—do is push their clients toward a certain type of birth based on their own beliefs or philosophies. Doulas undeniably grew out of the natural childbirth movement and are still strongly associated with it, but Simkin hopes they don't remain stuck there.

"At the very beginning, there was no doubt that we were there more for people who wanted a natural birth," said Simkin. "And medical people were totally entrenched [in their position]."

Simkin admits that her own emphasis on "natural," crucial in the cultural moment and context of women wanting to reclaim control from the medical establishment, was shortsighted. It took a particularly dramatic situation for her to abandon her position on medicated birth. She recalled a client with whom she was paired by the Washington State Department of Health as part of a program for low-income pregnant women.

"I called her on the phone and the first thing she said was, 'I don't want you talking me out of an epidural,'" Simkin said. She agreed, but confessed that she secretly thought, "Of course I will."

When Simkin met with her client in person, the first thing the woman did was insist again on having an epidural. As they talked, Simkin learned that the expectant mother was living in a shelter, having recently fled from an abusive husband. The woman told Simkin that she simply wanted a day without pain.

"I was converted immediately," she said.

As proponents of "natural" childbirth move away from absolute beliefs and toward a middle ground, members of the medical establishment seem to be doing the same. In 2014, the American Congress of Obstetricians and Gynecologists published a paper acknowledging that the national rate of Cesarean birth—one in three women in 2011—was too high, and that the tools long used by the "natural" birth community have an important role to play in bringing the rate down.

"Published data indicate that one of the most effective tools to improve labor and delivery outcomes is the continuous presence of support personnel, such as a doula," the paper states.[5] Currently, a small but growing number of hospitals around the country offer, along with obstetric care, in-house doula programs.[6]

But there is also another profound effect of labor support that can be summarized without any obstetric and clinical terms: Women with support have less negative feelings about childbirth. They are happier.[7]

These positive results are sometimes referred to as "the doula effect." While many nurses provide great care for their patients, favorable outcomes are higher when a woman is supported by someone she chooses herself, and when that person reports to no one but her.

There is a steadily increasing number of working doulas, but still only 6 percent of women who give birth in the United States use one.[8] Like farmers' markets and purchasing organic locally grown vegetables, which have captured our cultural imagination and become a way of life in wealthier, more progressive communities but account for less than 1 percent of agriculture sales in the country, easy and affordable access to doula support remains out of reach to most people.[9]

Doula services are rarely covered by insurance policies and people must pay hundreds, sometimes thousands, of dollars out of pocket for them. Outside densely populated urban areas, doulas are harder to come by. Perhaps it is not specifically a doula that every pregnant woman needs access to, but simply someone who is willing to take it upon herself to care for her.

In a study conducted by researchers at Rutgers University in 2006, low-income pregnant women at a hospital in New Jersey were asked to choose a female friend or family member to act as their support person during labor. These "lay doulas" were given four hours of training over the course of two, two-hour sessions. Even with just this small amount of training, results were clear: mothers who had these doulas had significantly shorter labors—by more than one hour—than those who did not.

"Information about the benefit of a female support friend should be dispensed at the first prenatal encounter and reinforced at each visit," the study concluded. "The empowerment a prenatal program such as this could provide may be especially important for low-income women . . . [and] may continue past the actual process of birth."[10]

This study is more than ten years old. We have known for over a decade that simply encouraging women to have a dedicated support person present during their labor could have lasting, affirming effects. Imagine how many more families could be helped by implementing this knowledge about the importance of care through formal programs.

*

We use the word "care" all the time. *Take care*, we say when we part ways or hang up the phone. *Take care*, we type as a sign-off on our e-mails. The *Oxford Dictionary* defines care as "the

provision of what is necessary for the health, welfare, mainte-
nance, and protection of someone." Pregnancy and birth are
handled through our country's health-care system—one in
which the "care" part can feel like an afterthought.

Until the Affordable Care Act was passed in 2010, 88 percent of individual plans did not cover maternity care.[11] It was
considered a "pre-existing condition" that could be excluded
from, or charged a much higher rate for, coverage. Under the
ACA, women's health services including maternity care and
birth control are listed in the ten essential health benefits that
all insurance plans are required to cover. Recent attempts
to repeal the legislation and cut Medicaid, which provides
health care to lower-income people, threaten this. The reduc-
tion of Medicaid would mean no maternity care for two million women—half of all women who give birth annually in
the United States.[12]

Caregiving is the fastest-growing occupation in the United
States, yet we barely speak about it.[13] We forget or gloss over
the fact that care is the backbone of our society and economy.
No one makes it earth-side, or through the helplessness of
infancy and childhood, without it. Nearly one in four new
mothers in America return to work just two weeks after giving birth—but no parent of any gender can return to the
workforce without some form of child care.[14]

Though they may be flawed and costly, we do have systems
in place that provide care. By guaranteeing maternity services
for all, we could begin to alleviate some of the unnecessary
stress and trauma that so many people experience during pregnancy and childbirth. But we shouldn't stop there. By looking

forward and focusing our efforts on creating truly inclusive care—care that supports all birth choices as well as underserved populations—we could create even better systems.

According to 2013's "Listening to Mothers" report, the only national survey of its kind that asks new mothers about their experiences with maternity care, nonwhite women are far less likely to access prenatal care than white women and experience more complications and a range of less favorable obstetrical outcomes.[15] (The survey, which has been published three times since 2002, was the first to systematically ask basic questions at the national level about the American maternity care system. Again, we didn't start doing this until 2002.) ACOG now acknowledges the need to recruit healthcare providers from more racial and ethnic groups to better serve an increasingly diverse group of patients.

Health-care providers are also beginning to acknowledge the number of survivors who, in giving birth, are forced to reckon with past experiences of sexual abuse. One out of every six women in America has been the victim of rape or attempted rape, and every year over sixty thousand children become victims of sexual abuse.[16] These traumatic memories lodge themselves in the body, beyond the reach of language, and can easily be triggered and reawakened during the physical intensity of pregnancy and birth. They undoubtedly contribute to birth being an excessively traumatic event for so many.

In 2004, Penny Simkin and Phyllis Klaus published *When Survivors Give Birth*, a resource for providers to care for mothers who have been victims through their pregnancy, birth, breast-feeding, and postpartum experiences. She and Klaus self-published the book, which has been reprinted eight times since, demonstrating that survivors have always given birth, even if health-care providers have been remiss to recognize them.

Simon Ellis, the certified nurse midwife, made a point to learn about trans reproductive care because throughout their own medical training, care of trans and gender nonbinary people was never included in any curriculum.

Ellis believes there are profound similarities between pregnancy and gender transition—two things that they have direct experience with. Both are temporary states of being that move you toward a future that, in most cases, is desired. Both require that your body be taken over by hormones and changed in ways that are both wondrous and frightening. The way that people look at you as a result of these physical changes will dramatically change, and the way that people interact with you—what they say you are allowed to do or should or should not do—will flip completely.

The forty-plus weeks of pregnancy and childbirth—going from not pregnant to pregnant and then, suddenly, from pregnant to not pregnant again—is a decidedly long and transformative process. As with birth, the binaries are extreme and bookmark the experience, but we spend most of our time in the middle. While we are there, we should exist as comfortably as possible. Care can be the buffer that supports us and fills in the gaps.

Care is vital to society but also an engine for other things:

decency, empathy, affection, love. We see it with our babies, where care is an obligation that begins at birth, before love can even be reciprocated. That care is expected makes it no less important; in fact, that's the whole point.

I'm grateful that I feel good about my birth experience, and I know that my perspective is in no small part the result of the care that I received. It is what others—the nurses, my doctor, the ob-gyn, the anesthesiologist, my husband, my doula—did for me. They took care of me. I needed them to, and I literally might not have survived without them.

In my case, despite excellent care, none of the expected improved obstetrical outcomes turned out to be true. My labor was long and grueling, and I ended up in surgery. But the emotional and psychological effects of being well supported made all the difference.

Sometime in the middle of the night, the nurse who put that pillow under my arm finished her shift and went home. I never saw her again. The rawness of my birth recedes into softer memories. But she left an indelible impression on me, a type of regard and empathy that will never be forgotten. It set me down a path—one strewn with uncertainty, leaking wounds, cracked nipples, and self-doubt—armed with a certain amount of faith in myself, in others. Faith that we could do it.

"Why can't we guarantee that a woman always feels well cared for?" Penny Simkin asked at one point during our conversation. "All we need is a human being. And she doesn't have to be a rocket scientist."

CHAPTER 7

MOTHER'S MILK

To produce breast milk, mothers melt their own body fat. Are you with me? We dissolve parts of ourselves, starting with gluteal-femoral fat, a.k.a. our butts and thighs, and turn it into food for our babies.

Breasts are complicated and fascinating organs. Out in the world, most of us hoist them up in bras, molding them into desired shapes under our clothing. At home, we let them hang out and rest, unencumbered. Some days they sit so buoyant, lovely, and proud, it's hard not to admire them. Other days, they feel so sensitive that a breeze makes them tingle or ache with pain, and we wish we didn't have to live with them at all.

Unlike our well-stocked ovaries and already beating hearts, or the living skin that envelops us at birth, breasts are not organs we're born with. Rather, they're something we acquire over time.

"You come into the world with a nipple and lots of potential: Some cells behind the nipple that, given the right hormonal stimulation, will grow and become a breast," wrote Dr.

Susan Love in 1990 in her now-classic women's health tome, *Dr. Susan Love's Breast Book.*[1]

Breasts have only one functional purpose: to make food for our offspring. Amid the sexualized images of breasts that abound in our culture, it can be hard to remember this. But breasts exist for babies first—any adult enjoyment or appreciation is secondary. Breasts can only fulfill their true calling through pregnancy. If they've never produced milk, they simply haven't reached full biological maturity (though they can still play a part in a happy and fulfilling life).

Of course, your breasts don't care whether or not you actually want to have a baby, end up giving birth, or decide to breast-feed a baby. They simply follow your lead and, when called upon, do their best to meet expectations. Sometimes they are successful; sometimes they are not.

Mature breasts are composed of adipose tissue (a.k.a. fat); stroma, the beautifully named network of ligaments and connective tissue; clusters of milk-producing alveoli cells; and a series of ducts to transport milk. Hundreds of alveoli cells gather into grapelike bunches called lobules, and groups of these lobules come together to form a lobe. The average breast is made up of twelve to twenty lobes, which are spread throughout the breast like the petals of a flower.

Milk ducts act as plumbing, transporting milk from their respective lobes. These ducts meet up, and milk from various lobes mix together and continue traveling to the nipple, where the liquid can exit the body. (Upon lactating, many women, myself included, are surprised to discover that there is not just one hole in the nipple, but six or seven.)

During monthly menstrual cycles, estrogen and progesterone stimulate the growth of more milk ducts and alveoli
cells. Woven amid all the lobes and stroma are also nerves, as
well as lymph and blood vessels, all of which are affected by
breast changes. The creation of new chambers and pathways
rearrange the structure of each breast, leading to the tenderness, lumpiness, swelling, and pain that many women experience as symptoms of premenstrual syndrome (PMS). If no
egg is fertilized, the uterine lining is shed, and breasts return
to their normal state. And then the whole cycle begins again.

Breasts are shape-shifters, constantly changing throughout
our lives. Before we have children, we may notice the monthly
fluctuations—heavy one day, smaller the next, weirdly sensitive another. For many women, it's precisely these sensations
that are the earliest signs of pregnancy. When we are pregnant, our breasts begin to change almost immediately, as hormones take their work to the next level. In the earliest weeks,
alveoli begin to expand, forming many distinct lobules that
increase breast volume from the inside.

Your breasts extend from your collarbone down to your
lower ribs and from your armpits to the middle of your chest.
When the hormones of pregnancy begin to do the work of preparing your body for motherhood, your overall blood volume
and flow increase. All of this causes your breasts to widen and
shift. By the end of the second month of pregnancy, breasts
can be noticeably bigger. At the end of pregnancy, breasts
may even be double their pre-pregnancy weight.

All these changes happen in preparation for lactation, which
is essentially the transmutation of blood into milk. Prolactin,

a hormone produced by the pituitary gland in the brain, compels alveoli cells to draw sugars, proteins, and fat from a mother's blood so that these macronutrients can be used as the building blocks of breast milk. Christians are taught that Jesus Christ once turned water into wine. Around the world, women's bodies perform a similar miracle, every hour, every day.

*

Before and after giving birth to my daughter, I was inundated with urgent directives from well-meaning, very insistent health practitioners, parenting book authors, mommy bloggers, journalists, and opinionated strangers that "breast is best." Barely anyone mentioned formula. The message was clear: in order to be a "good" mom, I had to breast-feed. I fell in line.

Studies show that breast-feeding leads to better overall health outcomes for children, which is why the World Health Organization (WHO), the United Nations International Children's Emergency Fund (UNICEF), the American Academy of Pediatrics (AAP), and the American Academy of Family Physicians (AAFP) all recommend that babies be exclusively breast-fed for a minimum of six months.[2] These organizations also suggest that breast-feeding continue, along with the introduction of appropriate solid foods, for at least one year, while WHO and UNICEF urge breast-feeding for two years or more.

Those outcomes, though, are relative: a premature infant

in a neonatal intensive-care unit or a baby growing up in a rural Ethiopian village with a high rate of infectious disease and no access to clean water will benefit significantly more from breast milk over artificial milk, a.k.a. formula, as compared to a healthy, full-term baby born in a modern American hospital.

Other research also suggests that breast-fed babies score higher on IQ tests later in life and have lower rates of childhood obesity than their formula-fed counterparts.[3] I understand why some parents find these statistics compelling, but when it came to my decision about how to feed my child, the results of a toddler IQ test or body mass index measurement didn't factor into my thinking.

More compelling to me were the facts about breast milk as it related to my daughter's health: It contains all the vitamins and nutrients a baby needs in her first six months of life; and it contains germ- and disease-fighting substances that help protect a baby from illness.[4] Oh, and also: *The nutritional and immunological components of breast milk change every day, according to the specific, individual needs of a baby.* Not nearly enough information is provided by doctors, lactation counselors, or the Internet about this mind-blowing characteristic of milk. I only found out when, weary after ten months of breast-feeding, I was looking for reasons and motivation to keep going.

Outside these health benefits, one of the biggest appeals of breast-feeding was what I believed to be its relative simplicity. It required nothing more than my body. My daughter latched easily at the hospital, which felt like a gift after such a long and hard labor and delivery. I was lucky. She nursed eagerly and freely, which made it simple for me to appreciate my body and stay committed to breast-feeding.

For my friend Giulia, whose baby was born the same week as mine and with whom we shared part-time child care, things didn't go as smoothly. Her son had trouble latching on from the beginning. After several weeks of lactation consultations and a visit to a craniosacral therapist, she eventually settled on a combination of pumping and formula feeding. It was disappointing, she told me, but I could also sense her relief, especially when, at the end of a workday, she got to sit down on the couch and watch her husband, Esteban, lovingly feed their son.

For another mother, Lauren, breast-feeding went great . . . until it didn't. Her goal—to breast-feed for one year—was informed partly by the fact that her own mother breast-fed her for twenty months. Like me, she had heard "over and over again how great breast milk was, and in the hospital, no other choice (i.e., formula) was presented as legitimate."

Breast-feeding, she said, "made me feel special because I was the only person who could provide that for my baby." But, she added, "I saw that power go both ways when I became unable to breast-feed after doing so successfully for about five months. It was torture."

Before I gave birth, I naively thought that breast-feeding required less time and equipment than formula feeding. But when I returned to office work, I learned that breast-feeding also entailed the time-consuming, painstaking, accessory-heavy (and often corrosively boring) reality of breast pumping. Every day I lugged to work a bag containing a cooler case, an ice pack, and a breast pump—complete with long plastic tubes, a pair each of bottles, caps, screw-on connectors, breast shields, valves, and membranes. I hooked myself up to it two times a day for almost half an hour each time, then rinsed each part out dutifully in the bathroom sink. (One day, under deadline and breasts painfully engorged, I made the maddening discovery that without the membranes—flimsy, inconsequential-looking, dime-size rubber flaps—the whole operation falls apart and no milk can be pumped from your breasts.)

For many mothers, pumping becomes akin to a second (or third) job. In fact, the greatest cost of breast-feeding, which is invisible to most people besides parents, is time (and, oh, bodily autonomy). For working mothers, making the time to leave their duties multiple times a day presents a significant challenge—especially at a time when they may need flexibility to arrive a few minutes late or leave a few minutes early because of child care needs. The lost wages incurred by time spent pumping and nursing is real. In fact, one report estimates that the monetary value of the time spent breast-feeding during the first six months adds up to $14,250.[5]

I made the choice to breast-feed around the same time I was offered a full-time job writing about food at a newspaper. Every morning at seven a.m., I nursed my daughter. At the office, I pumped milk twice a day, once in the morning and once in the afternoon. When I came home around five p.m., we nursed, and then at seven p.m., we nursed again before she went to bed. A few nights a week, I went out to dinner for work. My husband fed her a bottle and I pumped when I got home.

For six months straight, even when my daughter would sleep through the night, I woke up every night at three a.m. and pumped milk for half an hour in order to keep up a supply that made it possible for me to be away from her a few extra hours here and there. (Three a.m. is possibly the darkest, loneliest, and most quiet hour of the night, but I had the reassuring, rhythmic sound of my pale-yellow breast pump to keep me company.)

For more than a year of my life, there wasn't one minute when I wasn't thinking about, writing about, eating, or producing food.

*

Food points to who we are as animals—human beings with a fundamental need for nourishment, survival—but also to who we are as people: individuals with families, histories, stories, preferences, cravings. Every day, calories, nutrients, and even clues about the culture I live in flowed, dripped, leaked, and squirted out of my boobs, staining my clothes and making my skin sticky. And every day, I wondered what exactly went into the miraculous substance that was sustaining my daughter.

"People tend to underestimate what [breast] milk is," said Katie Hinde, a biologist and associate professor at the Center for Evolution and Medicine at the School of Human Evolution and Social Change at Arizona State University. She also runs the very funny, highly informative, and deeply nerdy blog *Mammals Suck . . . Milk!*

"That's in part because you go to the store and there's an entire aisle dedicated to buying milk that is literally a homogenized, standardized food. It leads us to take mother's milk for granted."

Hinde began studying mother's milk—a substance that is simultaneously food, medicine, and signal—in the late 1990s because, as she put it, "I had a lot of questions and there weren't any answers in the [academic] literature."

At the time, most research on human milk examined the benefits of breast-feeding versus formula feeding, but Hinde wasn't interested in that debate. She was interested in exploring the complexities of human milk, which has been around for hundreds of millions of years, through an evolutionary lens. She was curious how it might improve people's health and well-being now.

"If we think of an organism as a complex suite of adaptations that reflect ancestral environments, and any number of compromises, then we can understand: Why is milk the way it is? What does it do?" said Hinde. "These are the questions I would stay up late thinking about. At the time that I started my dissertation in 2002, nobody was really doing it. There were no answers."

Against the advice of her academic mentors, Hinde persisted. Since then, mother's milk has become a topic of interest in both anthropology and human biology. Right now, researchers like Hinde—a group that includes evolutionary biologists, dairy scientists, microbiologists, anthropologists, and food chemists—are examining human milk, and the more closely they look, the more complexities they find.

Nutritionally, breast milk is a complete and perfect food, an ideal combination of proteins, fat, carbohydrates, and nutrients. Colostrum, the thick golden liquid that first comes out of a woman's breasts after giving birth (or sometimes weeks before, as many freaked-out moms-to-be will tell you) is engineered to be low in fat but high in carbohydrates and protein, making it quickly and easily digestible to newborns in urgent need of its contents. (It also has a laxative effect that helps a baby pass its momentous first poop, a terrifying, black, tar-like substance called meconium.)

Mature breast milk, which typically comes in a few days after a woman has given birth, is composed of 3 to 5 percent fat and an impressive list of minerals and vitamins: sodium, potassium, calcium, magnesium, phosphorous, and vitamins A, C, and E. Long-chain fatty acids like DHA (docosahexae-noic acid, an omega-3 fatty acid) and AA (arachidonic acid, an omega-6 fatty acid)—both critical to brain and nervous-system development—also abound in mother's milk.

The principal carbohydrate in breast milk is lactose, a sugar that provides copious calories and energy to fuel babies' relentless, round-the-clock growth. (No, new parents, you are not hallucinating—your baby did just grow out of her pajamas sometime in the middle of the night.) Other sugars are also present, including some 150 oligosaccharides (there may be even more—scientists are really just beginning to understand them) and complex chains of sugars unique to human milk (I repeat: unique to human milk). These oligosaccharides can't be digested by infants; they exist to feed the microbes that populate a baby's digestive system, which are a critical part of her microbiome.[6] The human microbiome is a combination of bacteria unique to each of us that goes on to help us deal with infection, train our immune systems, and help process the food we eat. Microbes far outnumber our own cells, and they populate all the parts of our bodies.

And speaking of microbes, there are a ton of them in breast milk. Human milk isn't sterile—it's very much alive. Much like yogurt, naturally fermented pickles, and kefir—foods that help to keep our digestive systems functioning properly—breast milk is filled with beneficial microbes. So mother's milk contains not only the bacteria necessary to help a baby break down food but the food for the bacteria themselves to thrive. A breast-feeding mother isn't keeping one organism alive—but actually hundreds of thousands of them.

The flavors of breast milk are as dynamic as a mother's diet. Like a glass of red wine, breast milk has a straightforward color and appearance, but it possesses subtleties in flavor that reflect its terroir—the mother's body. And it turns out that like any great dish of food, mother's milk holds a variety of aromas, flavors, and textures.

In the 1970s, researchers at the University of Manitoba obtained samples of breast milk from lactating women and had them evaluated by a trained panel for taste, quality of sweetness, and texture. The researchers noted variations across samples in all categories, most notably the milk of a woman who had recently eaten spicy food, whose milk was described by tasters as being "hot" and "peppery."

The flavors of food ingested by breast-feeding mothers—kimchi, broccoli, mint, blue cheese—are infused into their milk and, in turn, tasted by their babies. Based on her research, Julie Mennella of the Monell Chemical Senses Center in Philadelphia has suggested that these early breast-milk experiences help infants develop their own personal taste preferences, as well as increase their appreciation of the flavors they are first exposed to via mother's milk.

My job allowed me to explore the diversity of Seattle's food scene, and, through my breast milk, my baby was able to sample it as well. I love the idea that even before her first encounter with solid food, her taste buds had already begun telling her that she was part of a city filled with the cuisines of many nations, a household that supports local farmers, and a Filipino family with an abiding love of pork and fermented shrimp paste. I'll never know for sure how these early exposures impacted her palate, but I like to think that it's more than a coincidence that soon after she began dabbling in solid foods, she eagerly scarfed down pork ribs smoked by her grandfather, roasted zucchini from a local farm, lechon and bagoong at a Filipino pop-up dinner, wild Neah Bay king salmon, and deep-fried hush puppies.

Just as exciting as the possibility that breast milk may have helped my daughter develop a healthy appetite, though, is the reality that it helped her live a healthier life in infancy. And that without my knowing it, my milk adapted itself to her needs with every feeding.

Studies show that breast-feeding is good for a baby's immunological health: breast-fed babies have lower instances of colds and viruses.[7] And when they do get sick, breast-fed babies are often able to recover quickly because their mother's body produces the specific antibodies needed to quell their infection. This idea—that my body could tailor-make medicine for my child like a kind of compound pharmacy—was so mind-blowing to me that I'd find myself pondering it as I pumped or nursed late at night. I wondered: how exactly was my body able to write my daughter a prescription for her illness without a diagnosis?

When I asked Hinde, she paused, looked straight through the Skype interface of her computer and directly into my eyes/soul, then said: "If I tell you, you can't unknow it. Are you sure you want to know?" (My answer: yasssssss.)

According to Hinde, when a baby suckles at its mother's breast, a vacuum is created. Within that vacuum, the infant's saliva is sucked back into the mother's nipple, where receptors in her mammary gland decipher it.[8] This "baby spit backwash," as she delightfully described it, contains signals, information about the baby's immune system—including any infections it may be fighting. Everything scientists know about physiology indicates that this baby backwash is one of the ways that breast milk is able to adjust its immunological composition.[9] If the mammary gland receptors detect the presence of pathogens, or germs, they compel the mother's body to produce the corresponding antibodies to fight them. Those antibodies are then passed through breast milk and back into the baby's body, where they target the infection.

At the same time that it is medicine, breast milk is also a private conversation between mother and child. When my daughter lacked words, breast-feeding made it possible for her to tell me exactly what she needed. The messages we sent each other were literally made of ourselves, and they informed us about what was going on in our lives at that very moment.

Mother's milk informs babies of not just the present but also the past. Returning to the maternal fat-melting thing, Hinde explained that mothers who are vegetarians in adulthood, but ate meat as teenagers, have stored fatty acids that are specific to animals. When they mobilize that fat to produce breast milk, their babies receive those nutrients.

"You have information about your whole life span that could be in your milk," said Hinde. "Milk is telling the baby about the world its mother has lived in."

Breast milk also plays a role in regulating a baby's circadian rhythm. Human babies aren't born with any concept of time, and some even seem to prefer a nocturnal schedule. Breast milk helps them to understand certain hours from other hours, night from day.

"Milk is so incredibly dynamic," said Hinde. "There are hormones in breast milk, and they reflect the hormones in the mother's circulation. The ones that help facilitate sleep or waking up are present in your milk. And day milk is going to have a completely different hormonal milieu than night milk."

Breast milk also holds the potential to address health disparities that exist in our society.

"Breast-feeding is one of the key public-health interventions that we can actually do," said Hinde. "Because we know that a lot of our metabolism, neurobiology, and immune function are shaped in huge ways by it—and that these have lifelong influences on how our bodies function."

We know that breast-feeding can help children avoid problems that manifest later in life, like type 2 diabetes and high cholesterol. We also know that black people are 2.2 times more likely than white people to develop type 2 diabetes, while Native Americans are 2.8 times as likely.[10] Black and Native American people have the two lowest initiation rates of breast-feeding of all racial and ethnic groups in the United States.[11]

There's another facet to breast milk that goes beyond benefitting the mother or the baby. Recently, researchers discovered that pluripotent stem cells, which are the highly valued stem cells that have the ability to form any of the more than two hundred different types of cells found in adult human bodies, are present in breast milk.[12] The only other place these cells have been found is in embryonic tissue.

"There are lots of ethical issues with [testing on] embryonic stem cells," said Hinde. "But breast milk could become a source of stem cells that can potentially be turned into any cell in the human body. There's huge potential for regenerative medicine."

And while science is a very long way off from being able to engineer and grow replacement tissue for people with degenerative diseases, breast milk offers a viable option for future studies.

*

I breast-fed because I wanted to and because my body cooperated with my wishes. I was able to continue breast-feeding because I have a supportive husband, a mother who watched her infant granddaughter three days a week for free, and a workplace that allowed me to exercise all of my breast-feeding rights as laid out by the Affordable Care Act. (For the record, mothers, you are entitled to: a breast pump, reasonable break time to express breast milk for one year after your child's birth each time you experience the need to express milk, and a place to pump, other than a bathroom, that is shielded from view and free from intrusion from coworkers and the public.)

But some mothers do not have family support and cannot afford to work and provide for child care during working hours. Other mothers might have financial security but work long hours or travel frequently, making nursing a near impossibility. And some mothers are met with resistance when they exert their Affordable Care Act–supported rights in the workplace.

According to the CDC, 75 percent of American mothers start out breast-feeding, but after six months, only 13 percent of babies are exclusively breast-fed.[13] Right now, we lack the societal, institutional, and cultural support structure to help mothers meet their breast-feeding goals. If we're telling women that they should breast-feed exclusively for six months, then we should give them—at minimum—the same amount of paid family leave. Seemingly everything about breast-feeding, which for the first few months easily takes up eight hours a day, is at odds with holding down full-time work. We do little to make it easier—or even viable—for mothers in the

trenches, pumping away in cramped offices and broom clos-
ets, working multiple jobs, forking over significant portions
of income to day care, and, yes, tired and close to the breaking point, cursing their own desire to continue feeding their
children their milk, to stick with it.

But there are also lots of other reasons why people stop
breast-feeding—some don't enjoy it, some are looking for a
more equal child care arrangement with their partner, and
some may just be too exhausted to continue their baby's feeding schedule. For people who present themselves in a less traditionally feminine way or who fall outside the gender binary,
breast- and chest-feeding can bring unwanted attention to a
part of their body that causes them stress. And some, like
Lauren, find that suddenly their bodies are no longer producing the same amount of milk.

The pressure to continue breast-feeding—despite the obvious fact that she simply was not making as much milk as
her daughter needed—exacerbated the postpartum anxiety
Lauren was experiencing.

"It was just this vicious cycle," she said. "I was having issues
breast-feeding because I was so anxious, and then I became
even more anxious every time I fed her and she would fuss,
cry, and pull herself away from me. It was so heartbreaking."

Lauren reached out to her doctor and several lactation con-
sultants, none of whom ever advised her that switching to formula was an acceptable option. "When I brought it up, they
said something along the lines of, 'If you decide to do that,
that's your choice.' I don't think they recognized that, at this
point, I really needed permission to stop breast-feeding."

(Despite this, Lauren's visit with one lactation counselor was beneficial in another important way. After screening her for postpartum depression, the counselor recommended she see a psychiatrist. Her recognition of the issue, which Lauren was not fully aware of, helped her get the treatment she needed.)

Even though she believed breast-feeding was still the best food for her daughter, Lauren eventually began using formula.

"[Breast milk] is the optimum food for babies. I know that's true, but there is a disconnect between how much the medical community is pushing breast-feeding and the American lifestyle," she said. "[My daughter's] well-being was linked to mine very strongly. I think we both would have benefitted a lot from me being more relaxed."

Even if the United States were to suddenly, magically offer breast-feeding mothers all the support they need, it's still unrealistic that every baby will be breast-fed. It doesn't mean we should give up—but it does mean that we should be asking: Are the millions of babies who drink formula multiple times a day getting the best possible formula? How can we make sure that all children, no matter how they are fed, get optimum nutrition?

Throughout its history, with the help of scientific research, we have consistently developed better formula. Since the late 1800s, manufacturers have added wheat flour, replaced animal fat with vegetable oils, and added specific vitamins and minerals such as iron, as well as amino acids.[14] Formula is now fortified with the omega-3 fatty acid DHA, which helps with brain development. Formula is a highly regulated food. While the manufacturers' recipes vary, the FDA Infant Formula Act dictates that all formula meets rigorous testing standards and nutritional requirements.

More recent research has proven that, as Hinde said, milk is living and dynamic. It changes daily, even more frequently than that, because a baby changes daily. And so new information is directing scientists to develop formula that is more active and adaptable. Researchers are trying to find ways to make better use of proteins, to add the oligosaccharides that feed the microbiome.

The Nestlé BabyNes formula system, which includes six stages of formula capsules for different stages of a child's life up to thirty-six months, is available in a few countries around the world, including the United States. It requires a special machine (cost: $199) that brews formula à la a Keurig coffeemaker and the capsules are prohibitively expensive, but it exists—and is being refined.

Figuring out how to best feed your baby can be hard, and it doesn't necessarily come naturally. The early (and later) struggles are discouraging. They can feel insurmountable. Breast-feeding mothers need trained support to help them keep trying. But they also need to be told that, if they want to, they can stop.

There is no right or wrong, there is just what we decide. What feels right—what is safe, enjoyable, and worth it— is what is best for a family. And we are all just doing the best we can.

The standards we set for mothers, without real support, mean that very few women will ever meet them. And even then, we often still feel inadequate.

If we can't love or trust our bodies completely, might we at least be able to accept them, let go, and move forward with the rest of life?

*

My daughter was born under the gray blanket of Seattle's fall, but once she started eating solid foods, I came to think of her as a summer babe. She loves Washington's Yakima nectarines and cherries, as well as the Skagit Valley strawberries and blueberries of early summer. Her first tomato—a small, beautiful Sweet 100 plucked from our garden—was still sun-warm when she bit into it, squirting seeds and juice onto her clothing and face. She likes the taste of the Italian plums that our neighbor John lets us pick from his tree, purple as bruises, even more than I do.

Breast-feeding is an intense relationship but ultimately one that lasts only a short period of time. As she ate more (and then more and more and more), she breast-fed less and less. By the time we weaned, it was obvious that, though she still needed me, she needed just as much to be part of the world, to touch and smell and taste it to be fully alive.

But still I will never forget when, a few weeks after she began eating solid foods, she developed a 101-degree fever. She was miserable, unable to sleep, and uncharacteristically disinterested in eating even the beloved blackberries we picked from the brambles a few blocks from our house. So we nursed instead.

As I held her close, her body fiery and fragile, I tried to

picture her saliva entering my body, my mammary glands interpreting it, my body producing her medicine, my breasts giving some defense against what she was fighting. And while I understood that these things were happening, it didn't feel any different, just the same soft, familiar tickle of her tongue against my nipple.

From the moment my girl exited my body, I've understood that being her mother would be a lifelong process of separation, letting go. But in that moment, I pulled her closer. I leaned in, as though I might actually hear her body whispering to mine.

III

A NEW YOU

CHAPTER 8

WHAT THIS BODY MEANS

The days after my daughter's birth are a foggy jumble—physical and emotional exhilaration and exhaustion sutured together in a throbbing line across my abdomen, all of it stewed in regular doses of narcotics. But I will never forget one afternoon during her first week outside my body, when I held her as she screamed. She had been doing this for hours, inconsolable and unable to sleep. I was in a panic, simultaneously fearing that I could not do this, and that if I could not do this, surely we would both be dead soon. I pulled her away from my chest and looked at her face, crying and saying, "I'm sorry, I'm sorry, I don't know what to do."

And then I looked into her eyes.

She was looking straight at me, and yet she wasn't. At first her eyes seemed like those of a drunk person—technically alert, but in reality, nobody's home. Then I saw what was shooting out of the depths of her black pupils, from the back of her crimson throat, and every cell of her clenched body: terror. It was unmistakable. I could relate.

I realized she was even more afraid of this new reality than I was, that she had even less of an idea of what to do. As I held her, both of us scared and sobbing and screaming, my husband came into the room, a different sort of fear on his face. He took her from my arms, gently suggested that I lie down for a while, and backed out of the room slowly. I was embarrassed that he had seen me so unhinged, but I felt grateful nonetheless.

He and I were a team—a battered, sleep-deprived team, but still one that had been working well together for years. Now that we had a new team member, we had to figure out how to be there for each other, as well as for the tiny, helpless human we had just brought into the world.

When our team left the hospital, its rookie screaming in the back seat for the entire twenty-minute drive home, I was recovering from surgery and still very weak. The most basic movements—standing up, walking, using the bathroom, and climbing up and down stairs—required great effort. Cooking, which usually serves as the calming anchor of my days, felt like an impossibility. I was breast-feeding every two hours, and most of my other time was spent bouncing on an exercise ball, trying to soothe and shush my daughter to sleep.

I learned quickly that I needed my partner in the most basic ways. While I was held hostage on the couch, strapped into a My Brest Friend nursing pillow with an infant latched on to my body, I needed him to bring me a glass of water, some crackers, the remote control. I needed him to make me tea, fold my clothes, go outside and get the mail.

It felt like I was breathing through just one lung, like I only had the use of my right hand. He became my other hand. We tag teamed, subbing in and out constantly: I fed the baby, he burped her. He put her down, I picked her up. He changed the diaper, I threw it away. She spit up into my (unwashed) hair, he appeared instantaneously with a burp cloth to wipe away the curdled goo. I am aware how lucky I was to have this support; I know a lot of people do not.

Normally this level of dependency would have scared me. I would have fought it. I would have picked (seemingly un-related) fights about it. But I was too desperate to care about pride. Rather than reject his efforts to help me, I accepted my newfound vulnerability with gratitude.

In the first few weeks of our daughter's life, my husband became, as many partners do, a butler of sorts: retrieving burp cloths, fetching water, doing daily loads of laundry. These are essential tasks, but compared to the creation and mainte-nance of life, they are unglamorous and menial. He asserted his desire to do more "important" work by occasionally in-sisting that I rest while he took care of the baby, even when she seemed to only want or need me. Through the clouds of exhaustion, I couldn't see the ways he, too, was changing.

"I was willing to work at it for five hours even if you could do that in ten seconds," he told me later. "I really wanted to be able to soothe her, to calm her. I look back and realize it was silly, but I still did it."

As her mother, I had already done the lion's share of work getting her onto this earth; as her father, he just wanted to spend a few hours getting her to sleep. He and his daughter— their bodies, their scents, screams, skin, and stubble—had to figure it out for themselves, to forge their own relationship, without me.

*

Around the time our daughter turned two, she was fond of Eric Carle's book *The Very Hungry Caterpillar*, the story of a caterpillar that hatches out of its egg and spends the next week eating a massive amount of food, including four strawberries, an ice cream cone, a pickle, and one "nice green leaf." Healthy and fat, the caterpillar builds a cocoon to stay in for a couple of weeks. On the final page of the book it emerges transformed—a brilliant, beautiful butterfly.

My family became deeply acquainted with this caterpillar and its activities. For more than a month, we read the book every morning, afternoon, and evening, usually a minimum of four times per sitting. Each time we got to the end, our daughter would turn to us and say, sweetly but firmly, "Again."

As we learned a new level of patience, she learned language. She relished saying words she already knew out loud: "Pop!" "Sausage!" "Watermelon!" Gradually, she grasped the pronunciation and meaning of the word "cocoon." I watched as her constantly churning brain began to understand that this was the place where the caterpillar did its remarkable work of metamorphosis, changing its form into a completely different one.

Of course, my daughter didn't understand the actual nuances of the caterpillar's metamorphosis: inside its cocoon, it releases enzymes that dissolve most of its tissue into a soupy mix of proteins, rearranges its anatomy, then develops into a new creature. But the excitement and beauty of the transformation—the butterfly's wings, their bright reds and blues and purples—was obvious. The appeal of this biological process is so powerful that humans can't help but ascribe spiritual, even miraculous, qualities to it.

Caterpillars may be the most famous and dramatic shape-shifters, but other animals—including we humans—constantly transform ourselves in subtle, but no less significant, ways. It's how we survive.

The slipper lobster is a wide, splayed-out crustacean that has ten legs but lacks the signature claws of its better-known relatives. Slipper lobsters hatch from eggs in the form of unique larvae called phyllosoma, which are transparent and so thin as to be nearly flat. Eventually the larvae become hard-shelled, bulky animals. But they begin life see-through, vulnerable, and almost cartoonish. They sport big eyes and hitch rides around the ocean on the backs of jellyfish.

As it matures, a lobster continues developing through a series of changes called molts. It outgrows its tough exoskeleton and must shed it in order to thrive. With each molt, its armor falls off to accommodate a new one that is forming underneath. Until that new shell hardens, though, the lobster is left tender and exposed. While they are susceptible to predators, it is also the only time that females are able to mate.

From a very young age, we teach our children to be awed by the changes in the natural world. Can we ever see our own changes with the same generosity and wonder?

Like other animals, we build protective shells around ourselves—habits, coping mechanisms, cynicism, stoicism— and they calcify and harden. We come to believe that this is who we are. But we are more than our defense mechanisms. All lives transform, and so must we.

When we brought our daughter home, she was all soft and squishy parts, as well as transparent desires. She was small, but her presence was huge. She brought both tremendous peace and disruption to our life. The forces came like a typhoon, wave after wave, alternately baptizing and wrecking us.

We brought her into our bed, a nearly holy space of close-ness and calm, where for weeks she slept in the center. We will-ingly placed a force we had no control over in between us. We were transfixed by her melodic coos and the adorable smiles she offered us in her sleep. We were undone by her abrupt awaken-ings and cries. There was a new, milky sweet intimacy to our shared space but also a loss of ballast and steady comfort.

My husband and I like our sleep. Aside from the first two years of our relationship, which we spent closing down bars because we never wanted to stop talking to each other, most evenings of the ten-plus years that we've been together have been planned around getting eight hours of rest. He likes to remind me that for most of his life he was "a legendary sleeper," falling asleep while in line at Six Flags Great America for a roller coaster, once on a moving sailboat in high wind.

Having a child destroyed that.

"Now if she makes the slightest peep—boom, I'm wide awake," he said ruefully. "The old sleep is gone."

For the better part of a decade, the primary purpose of

our bodies had been to give and receive pleasure to the other: through conversation, stimulation, food, movement, touch, sex. Now they were being used for a decidedly more practical, less romantic purpose: to keep us fed, clean, alive.

Four days after coming home from the hospital, I had a harrowing experience for which no one had prepared me: my first postpartum poop. (Whether you deliver vaginally or via C-section, you will be constipated after your birth. Not eating full meals during labor, taking painkillers, having your intestines moved around, causing gas and bloating, as well as having hemorrhoids and a torn-up perineum from pushing all make it difficult to move your bowels.)

After days of taking stool softeners and drinking prune juice, I finally felt the urge. I sat on the toilet for what felt like an eternity, making slow progress, needing to push, yet afraid to do so, lest all my digestive organs slip out of me. I had not pushed my eight-pound baby out of my body, but for a moment I thought that this is what it would have felt like. When it was finally over, weeping, I summoned my husband to the bathroom and asked him to do the previously unthinkable: to look directly at my asshole and make sure my insides weren't falling out. I wanted to be humiliated, and for him to be horrified by the situation, but oddly, neither of us was. My colon still in place, we went back about our business.

Just shy of six weeks postpartum, out of nowhere, I felt another strong urge: for sex. "Sexual" is probably the last word I would use to describe how I was feeling at the time, but I wanted badly to know that we could do it—that my body was still capable of giving me and my husband that kind of enjoyment. Thankfully, it was. But as I straddled him, my body issued a clear statement about its priorities. Just as I reached my first postpartum orgasm, breast milk sprayed— and I mean sprayed like a fire hose, not a garden hose, not a gentle trickle from a tap—out of both of my boobs, hitting our pillows, our headboard, and my husband's face.

Oxytocin is known as the "love hormone" because it produces a feeling of well-being and contentment during orgasm, birth, and breast-feeding. Or, in this case, a tangled, sticky web of these things. My body was declaring that the oxytocin it was producing was not in service of me or my desires. I watched in horror as my husband, stunned and slightly panicked, opened his mouth and moved his head side to side like a baby bird, trying in vain to catch all the liquid. I clamped my hands over my breasts and dismounted, mortified. This was not the kind of sex I wanted to be having.

In that moment, I understood that it was not just how our bodies related to each other that had changed but also how my body related to me. Becoming a mother, I took on a secondary role within it even as I was doing something that had nothing to do with my child. It was disorienting to exist as a shadow to my own yearnings, my body automatically prioritizing her needs ahead of mine. Her attachment to my physical being, it was telling me, was more urgent, more important than my own. I looked down at my body, trembling and satisfied, yet simultaneously deflated and empty. I did not recognize it, not in the slightest, though it was still the only home I'd known since the day I was born.

Before I became pregnant, I had worked hard to love, or

at least accept, my body. I had always suspected it was a little too round, dark, and much for this world, but by age thirty-six, I saw its beauty, appreciated its strength, learned to trust and listen to its particular thirsts and appetites. But in those weeks, months—years, really—immediately after giving birth, I didn't know how to feel about it.

It was months before I was truly interested in sex again. My husband never put any pressure on me, but, wanting to be a good partner and wanting to feel like myself, I was willing to go through the motions every now and then. But, as someone who enjoys having a partner take charge and use a little force, I was frustrated to find that my husband was reluctant to be anything but gentle with me. I didn't want to be treated as fragile, even though I undeniably was. Turns out it is pretty much impossible to convince someone to be aggressive toward you when you have a large abdominal wound and are prone to sobbing.

Pregnancy, with its attendant hormones and increased blood flow to her vulva and vagina, gave my friend Eve a surprising sexual boost. Her orgasms felt stronger and better ("even the most boring one was on par with my best ones before"), and she happily gave in to this temporary, heightened aspect of pregnancy.

"My body felt high, supercharged," she said. "Yes, achy and tired and napping, too, but also *really, really, really* alive."

But after her son's birth—which included painful back labor, as well as an emergency hospital transfer and C-section—she is still struggling to make sense of her sexual self and her physical relationship with her spouse.

"My body has been drenched with the same hormones, plus the prolactin," she said, referring to the other postpartum hormone that enables new mothers to produce breast milk. Prolactin has the opposite psychological effect of oxytocin; it creates a feeling of tension, of needing to be with or hold your baby.[1]

"I couldn't orgasm for months," she said.

She has always been a dominant sexual partner but said that now, "I can't feel that thing I need to feel to persuade someone to surrender to me, because I can't quite imagine someone looking at my body and assessing it as desirable enough to offer that to me."

"I am afraid to own a Body— / I am afraid to own a Soul— / Profound—precarious Property," wrote the poet Emily Dickinson. But the body, Dickinson concludes, is inescapable: "Possession, not optional." Post-pregnancy, our bodies are softer, uglier, scarier, more awe-inspiring, and more raw than they have ever been. But also never more useful or hardworking.

It was never my body's job to be perfect, just to keep me alive. I did not fully understand this until it was also what kept someone else alive.

In the early days of nursing my daughter, there was a popular song on the radio that seemed to follow me wherever I went: coffee shops, the grocery store, the car, and the dressing room at Target. It was an echo-y, spacy electronic dance music song—not the type of thing I'm usually into—by an English group called Disclosure. One morning, I finally tuned in to the lyrics as I drove to work: "Now I've got you in my space / I won't let go of you / Got you shackled in my embrace / I'm latching on to you."

My god, was this song written from the perspective of a nursing baby? The title of the song was "Latch." "Latch" is not an uncommon word, but if you have ever breast-fed or attempted to breast-feed, you know it is a word that, in the early days of your baby's life, will dominate nearly every conversation: *The baby needs to get a good latch. How's his latch? When the baby's lips are "flanged," then you'll know you've got a good latch. The baby needed formula because she was having problems with her latch.* Before I had a baby, I'd never heard the word used much. Afterward, I seemed to hear it thirty times a day, sometimes within the echo chamber of my own brain.

"If there are boundaries, I will try to knock them down," the British man on the radio/the baby in my mind sang. "I'm latching on, babe, now I know what I have found."

I understood that this was a love song (albeit a slightly creepy one) that should have made me think of my husband, but in my postpartum mind it was clearly written about me and my baby. The simplicity of its emotions made it possible for me to hear both the perspective of an infant and mother, as though the two were interchangeable.

The love I had for my baby felt more like all-consuming, irrational, romantic love than I would like to admit: the falling for, obsessiveness, and the fuzzy-chested, dizzying joy of getting to know her. And then there was the physical attachment that, while overwhelming and draining, was also somewhat addictive and unquenchable. I kissed her face, stroked her feathery hair, and inhaled her body's scent, taking long sniffs of the top of her sweet, musky head.

It was as if our bodies were merging all over again, and yet there was the knowledge that we were totally separate now. That while she depended on my physical body, she was not simply an extension of me. She was an individual, slowly revealing herself to me in snippets and flashes. There was both a thrill and a sting to the separation. Even as we celebrated each milestone of independence, there were moments that broke me: when she suddenly refused the comfort of my arms or ran to her father or grandmother before me.

What I couldn't fully appreciate then was the knowledge I have now: that being a mother means honoring the distinct people we have always been and recognizing that, as members of a family, we'll be finding our way apart and together, again and again, for a lifetime.

*

No pregnancy or parenting book or website or class prepared me for the regular seismic shifts—both physical and psychological—of parenting. It's not hard to imagine why. How do you instruct new parents, who are already working as hard as they can just to keep up with the demands each day brings, to also, in their spare time, lean into the utter obliteration of their previous selves?

If you were to ask a group of new parents how they're adjusting to their new reality, you'd be met with answers ranging from elation to anxiety. But among those responses, there would more than likely be a few suggestions of a sense of loss—over their old selves, their old lives. According to a study conducted at the University of California–Davis, parenthood delivers a serious blow to the self-esteem of both women and men.[2]

The researchers found that, just before childbirth, hopeful parents of both sexes experienced a boost in their self-esteem. But in the years after childbirth, mothers and fathers experienced a decline in positive feelings about themselves. (There was also evidence that mothers' self-esteem plummeted right after birth, suggesting that they are more impacted, whether from the initial stress of caring for a newborn or the hormonal drop-off experienced around the same time, than fathers.) The researchers followed the couples for five years, monitoring their moods and emotions. And in that time, they found no significant improvement in the parents' self-esteem.

How is self-esteem defined or measured? The psychologists who conducted this study correlated adult self-esteem with being good at what we do—mastering a set of skills, many of which are related to the work we do. The arrival of a baby gives us a whole new, arguably more important, job: parenting. And parenting, no matter how much we read up or prepare ourselves for it, is chaotic, trial-by-fire-type work. The job requirements—keeping a helpless, not fully developed person alive on no more than a few hours of sleep at a time, getting up close and personal with human excrement multiple times a day—are demanding. And even when you think you've mastered a new skill, your baby will quickly evolve her needs so that yesterday's accomplishments feel meaning-less today. Day after day, hour after hour, your infant will remind you how little you know about what you are doing. For people who are used to doing things well, this can be more than frustrating. It can start to feel like failure.

"Even though the birth of a child is generally considered a positive event," wrote the researchers in the kind of honest and detached tone that I could only ever aspire to, "it is still associated with numerous potentially taxing challenges, and these tangible negative aspects of parenthood may offset the more abstract positive characteristics of the event."

"A lot of my self-worth before came from extreme competence, from being able to juggle multiple things and do them all extremely well," said Eve, who thrived on achieving her career goals and organizing her family's finances and home life. But becoming a parent—a jagged labor, recovering from surgery, caring for an infant without adequate rest—forced her to surrender, to acknowledge that she couldn't take care of herself, work, and her household totally and independently.

"After the baby, I was doing just an adequate job, and I hated it," she said. "Becoming someone who does things acceptably well, but not notably well, is really hard on me."

Why don't we prepare parents for this reality? Why don't we talk openly about the fact that while there is much joy in becoming a parent, caring for a young child is also grueling, sometimes depressing work? That as we gain a new life, we also lose an old one?

How do we measure our own self-worth when our new self is barely recognizable? We cannot use the same values that applied to our lives before we were parents—being an ever-present friend or tireless worker, being stylish or the life of a party—when it is hard to sleep, find pants that fit, leave the house.

Caring for an infant is monotonous, constant, and physically demanding work. New parents should be regarded like endurance athletes or hard laborers. Your body acquires another layer of utility, albeit one besotted with emotion, and its willingness to do that is how we should regard it, first and foremost. The work is honorable; doing the work is beautiful.

*

During the early, messy days of my daughter's life, I found myself thinking a lot about my friend Marina. She got pregnant six years before I did, long before I had even considered having children. In the middle of her pregnancy, her relationship with the baby's father ended. He moved out, and she began making plans to give birth and raise their son on her own.

She wasn't entirely alone. A group of friends threw her a baby shower. I went to midwife appointments with her. Another friend stepped in to be her birth partner and was by Marina's side throughout labor and delivery. Her mother flew across the country soon after the baby was born and stayed with them for a few weeks, holding the baby, cleaning the house, taking care of her, and cooking the fiery northern Thai food that Marina grew up on. (Nearly ten years later, her mother still comes back regularly for weeks or months at a time to help raise her grandson.)

I am ashamed to admit that, until I had a newborn of my own and felt myself barely holding on to sanity and desperately needing a partner's support, it had never occurred to me just how hard it must have been for Marina. That's one thing about motherhood—often until it happens to you, you have no idea what it's like. Imagining what it is like feels irrelevant to daily life. I found myself wondering how the hell my friend got through those early months.

"Honestly, I don't know. I just decided to figure it out," she told me when, years later, I finally asked. She looked at me with wet eyes, her voice shaking. "It was hard."

Marina gave birth at home. A few hours later, her midwife left. And soon after that, much to her dismay, her birth partner left, too.

"I think [my birth partner] thought I just needed rest. She literally brought me a container of pasta salad, put it by the bed, and left," she said. "And after, all I could think was, 'This is when I really need you.'"

Marina spent the first few days in bed, sleeping and breastfeeding in an exhausted stupor, her baby boy by her side. Like anyone, she wondered if and how she would make it. But she had no one to distract her from those dark thoughts, and no one to help her when she felt overwhelmed by the job of caring for a newborn.

"I remember just lying in bed looking at him and thinking, 'What the fuck am I doing? Maybe I shouldn't be doing this. Maybe I should put him up for adoption,'" she said.

"I can't say that I thought about it for more than a day, but

I knew: This is the time. If I'm going to give him away or keep him, I need to decide now."

Her instincts took over. She found reserves and resources that she never knew existed inside herself and she pushed through. She's been drawing on those same resources to make it through each day since.

Not all of our relationships with mothers are marked by love. Some mothers are not capable of caring for us. And not every mother experiences an instant bond, which can make them feel inadequate and isolated. Parenthood throws you off your game, at least temporarily, and it changes the course of your life. That change can breed sadness, anxiety, sometimes resentment. Not everyone can overcome, or even recognize, those feelings.

Lauren felt anxious "pretty much all the time, constantly on edge." While she had been managing her anxiety well most of her adult life, the acts of caring for her daughter— worrying if she was getting enough sleep and enough to eat, specifically—kicked her anxiety into overdrive. It also triggered a deep depression.

"For weeks at a time, I was sleeping only an hour or two a night. My mind had become so dark," Lauren said of the transition that occurred. "I literally felt like I had nothing to live for and that I would never get better." Eventually, with her family's encouragement, she got treatment.

"I never would have believed that I would end up in a psychiatric hospital," she said. "If someone wanted to bet me a million dollars about it, I probably would have taken them up on their offer. But anyone can have a mental illness or become depressed."

Many of us experience dark moments and difficult periods, but not all of us have a support network and path out. It isn't anyone's fault if they don't. It's not hard to see how the obliteration of the self, without any support or acknowledgment of this shift, could break someone. Or how the need to survive could cause a mother to detach from her emotions.

Nearly a year after our daughter was born, my husband and I went out to dinner to celebrate our anniversary. As we sat there, martini glasses between our fingers, he asked me how I was feeling.

"Honestly," I told him, "that feels like an irrelevant question. I'm just doing stuff."

I was stunned to find that, as someone who spent most of her twenties writing down the subtle contours of every feeling in a journal and crying, I was now saying that feelings were irrelevant, an impediment to getting through each day. But it was true. It was easier and far more useful to talk about the things that needed to get done—grocery shopping, bill paying, taking out the garbage, feeding our daughter, getting her down for a nap—than the emotions I experienced while doing them.

I had been exposed for the beast I truly was; my primary concern was enduring. It was only after about eighteen months that the richness of life—a less debilitating sense of tiredness, being able to notice the changing of seasons—began to creep back in. Around the same time, our daughter started to be able to show us real affection. *I feel like I just came up for air*, I told a friend. *I didn't realize I had been drowning.* I began to feel like myself—or at least a more familiar version of myself—again. My husband and I started to catch glimpses of what it was like to be us, to spend time together, before we were parents. Any time we were able to go out for dinner or drinks alone, we made a rule that we couldn't talk about the baby. We tried our best to stick to it.

The effects of new parenthood on the relationship between partners have been studied by psychologists for decades—and the results have consistently shown that the quality of a couple's relationship declines once a baby comes into the mix. More recently, researchers at the University of Connecticut sought to understand why this happens. The results of their research indicate that it may have a lot to do with the expectations mothers and their partners have about the division of labor and child-rearing responsibilities.

Researchers found that couples who didn't discuss parenting chores and who is in charge of which task—"unexpressed and incongruent role expectations"—had more negative feelings about their relationships. In contrast, having similar beliefs about the need to share tasks—and being clear about who is responsible for what—helped couples maintain a happier relationship amid the chaotic banality of early parenthood.[3]

My husband and I did our best to prepare for the changes ahead. Just before I returned to office work, we sat down together and drew up a wholly unromantic list of chores and divided them equally between ourselves. Everything from taking out the recycling, making shopping lists, and cleaning the bathrooms was now assigned to one of us, taking into account not just our preferences but our abilities. For example, he took on the task of cooking breakfast every morning—something I love to do but could not do while sitting in a chair nursing a baby. We traded in spicy egg dishes for bowls of plain oatmeal.

Interestingly, the study also found that relationship satisfaction was affected only "marginally by whether partners' ideal division of role responsibilities matched the actual division of responsibilities." So, even if I was late scrubbing out the toilet bowl or pulling the massive tangle of my hair that slows down our shower drain, my husband at least appreciated my willingness to get on my hands and knees to do so. We decided how to divide the work, though we didn't necessarily stick to the plan. It was having the conversation in the first place that gave us a fighting chance.

Parenting is a 24–7 job; it never stops, and neither do the many tedious logistical negotiations that go along with it. Someone has to make sure there is clean laundry, food in the house, diapers. Chores are one thing, but there is also the domestic emotional labor of being tuned into a kid's ongoing needs—her evolving nap schedule, shoe size, nutritional requirements, the type of play and stimulation she requires. These tasks tend to fall on one partner and, in heterosexual couples, disproportionately on women. Sixty-four percent of all moms with preschool-age children work; mothers are the primary breadwinners in 40 percent of households with children under the age of eighteen. (This number is even higher for black moms, who, because of higher rates of single motherhood, are the primary breadwinners in 74 percent of house-holds.)[4]

Even with many women's feet firmly planted in the outside workforce, an extra level of sacrifice of mind and body is still expected.

*

One day while walking through the magazine section at my neighborhood library, I passed a copy of *Health* magazine (tagline: "Happy Begins Here") with Jillian Michaels on the cover. She was wearing blue panties and a striped sweater that was pulled up to reveal her taut stomach. "GET YOUR BODY BACK!" Jillian and her Slimdown Plan screamed at me. Silently, and without thinking, I walked past her, toward the cookbook section, middle finger raised.

I wonder why we need new mothers to look like we did be-fore we had babies. Why we push ourselves to "get our bodies back." My body will never go back to what it was; it's made a person, traveled to another dimension, and given birth to another world. The journey has left more than a few marks. I want to embrace that.

But as much as I want to celebrate my body and what it has accomplished, it is hard not to compare it to its old version. I still find myself wanting to fit into all my old clothes, to feel strong in familiar places, to recognize my physical form in a mirror, precisely because the rest of me—my internal world—still feels foreign and new. I sometimes get envious (and sometimes am filled with rage) when I see other mothers whose bodies aren't saddled with the same heft I have around my middle, or whose breasts seem unaffected by gravity. I try to remind myself that most of them are probably grappling with the same feelings that I am.

Eve, whose son is breast-feeding and more dependent on her body, is still mourning the loss of her old shape and wardrobe.

"Dresses are how I feel at home, normal. But you can't breast-feed in public in a dress," she told me. "Living in a world of wonky shirts and jeans and pants that don't fit a new lower belly makes me feel defeated. My new body also stole all my heels. My new feet only fit my ugliest clunky work shoes and some sneakers. I'm trying to remember that it's temporary."

We look externally to control what is inevitable, what is ordinary. Or maybe we look to the external as a way of giving order to the disarray inside us. Either way, physical changes are natural and they follow their own timeline. I think of the caterpillar, brown and soupy in its cocoon, awaiting its big moment. A world full of slow transformations. Coral, bleached of its colors by rising ocean temperatures, doesn't pretend to be unaffected by nature. Rocks, worn into smooth submission over years by tumbling water, don't deny what has happened to them.

Looking back I realize that, facing each other at the table every morning, my husband and I were like a pair of slipper lobsters, worn and tired as an old pair of shoes. Our former shells were falling off and new ones were forming, all while our bodies, more tender than ever, were showing us what we were capable of.

Our affection for each other was strengthened day by day. It acquired another layer—hard-won, animal, essential. I loved him more and more just for his stale-breathed, crusty-eyed existence. For showing up for me every morning. For making a humble bowl of warm sludge that gave our blurry days a place to begin.

The affection of a baby is no substitute—nor is it fair to expect that it will be—for the physical home of another adult body. Eventually, having taken months to recover from the fire hose incident, I was genuinely interested in having sex regularly again. We started feeling our way back to it. Sometimes sex was perfunctory. Sometimes sex was urgent and hot. Sometimes sex was soft and almost frightening in its intimacy. Just like it was before the baby. But there are moments, too, when our connection feels deeper, something primordial that was forged in gunk and muck when we crossed the line of parenthood from which there was no going back.

The other morning over breakfast, which he still makes for us most days, I told my husband about the slipper lobster. He laughed and we watched a YouTube video posted by a Japanese aquarium of one molting in a tank.[5] It was set to lighthearted polka-style music. At the end of its long, slow shimmy, the lobster finally wrests free of its shell. It pops up with surprising momentum and then falls backward onto its tail. It withdraws itself from that other body, just as we do after sex, and it sits for a moment, looking exhausted, satisfied, and spent, before it backs into a corner and curls up into itself.

"Yup. You're totally vulnerable," he said to the lobster on my computer screen, nodding and encouraging it as though they were friends. "You don't know where you're going, or what you're going to look like at the end of it all, but at least you're moving in a new direction."

CHAPTER 9

THE SEAT OF POWER

I was around eight years old when I found my parents' copy of *The Joy of Sex* hidden inside the built-in storage benches in their bedroom, the ones with the satiny green cushions that I liked to laze around on, reading and daydreaming. The cover of the book was timeless, simple, and white, but its pages were straight out of the 1970s: pencil drawings of a woman and man, armpits and pubic areas overflowing with dark hair, him with a mangy beard and chest hair peeking out of a barely buttoned shirt. They touched each other tenderly, caressing and exploring parts of human bodies that I had never seen before, doing things I couldn't even imagine.

My parents never talked to me about sex or vaginas or penises. Throughout my life I had been instructed never to touch my "pekadoodee" except to clean it vigorously. I knew that I should not be looking at this book, just as I knew I would be studying every page.

Nearly thirty years later, a similar, slightly illicit twinge ran through me when, while settling in to study for an anatomy class, I accidentally flipped my textbook open to the page with illustrations of the male and female pelvic floor. I gasped. At first glance, it was terrifying. The perspective of the drawings made it seem like I was lying on the floor looking upward, straight into someone's hairless, well-lit crotch as they squatted above my face. The flesh was cut away, exposing the muscles and fat underneath. There, spread wide and staring back at me, was the hole of the vagina, a set of anuses, and the underside of naked testes, stripped of their scrotums.

I stared for a few moments, shocked but soon mesmerized. What I saw was beautiful. Layer upon layer of muscles, an intricately woven basket of fibers, diagonal and horizontal lines in crimson, pink, and gray. And, in the center, muscle shapes that I had not seen before: not long, sinewy lines, but small circles stacked upon each other. On the female body, they formed a figure eight or, when I turned my head, the infinity symbol: eternity displayed unambiguously in my crotch.

Up until this moment, I had no idea this is what I look like. What we all look like.

For weeks after, just as I did with that copy of *The Joy of Sex*, I found myself creeping back to it. I studied the pictures, read the text: *bulbospongiosus, levator ani, the deep transverse perineal*. These are the muscles our bodies use to hold and remove waste, to support our organs, to reproduce. This is our seat of power: where we experience ecstasy and vulnerability, where we conceive, grow, and pass our children into the world.

And yet it's an area of our body that we are told very little about, even in pregnancy. Looking back at the forty weeks

I spent devouring books and dutifully paying attention in childbirth classes, I realize I had no clue what was actually happening to these parts of my body and what happened to them during and after birth.

Two years into my postpartum journey quest to vanquish persistent hip pain, I took a pelvic floor strengthening class. It was taught by a woman I happened to take a dance class with, who made a quick announcement one day that she would be offering it at a neighborhood yoga studio. Our class of five women was small and intimate, and as a way of breaking the ice, we introduced ourselves and talked about what had brought us there.

"I want to learn about this part of my body," I said, "to see if there is something I can do to help with the pain I'm feeling every day."

"I just want to not pee every time I run, which is the one thing I do just for myself every day," one woman said.

"I just want to not pee every time I laugh, because that is how I stay happy," said another woman.

It turned out we were all mothers, each of us trying to solve a problem we didn't fully understand, all wanting to learn about ourselves.

We rely on our pelvic floor for closure and control—to pee and poop and, perhaps more important, not to pee and poop until the time and location are right. We need these parts to be able to relax, too, so that when we crave stimulation and sex, we can open ourselves to these things. The pelvic floor is both an essential guardian and gateway, yet we are taught virtually nothing about its anatomy or function.

The muscles and organs of the pelvis—think of it as your "lower core," the area between your abdomen and thighs—are like the sanitation workers of the body. They whisk away waste and secrets, the evidence of our messy lives. They take materials to be recycled and composted, helping to nourish and regenerate the earth, allowing us to remain here for just a little longer. They come through our dark alleys, their work hidden and taken for granted. But as many children understand, including my daughter, who gleefully waves at her lifelong friend Mr. Rod as he comes down our alley in his big green truck every Wednesday, these workers are indispensable.

The foundation of the female pelvis is composed of two hip bones, which come together to form a deep bowl that is filled by the uterus, ovaries, bladder, urethra, vagina, and colon. The bones connect with the sacrum in the lower back and, in the front, they form a strong but flexible joint called the pubic symphysis. The symphysis is fused by cartilage that softens during pregnancy and birth to make more room for the baby's journey out of the womb.

Your pelvis also holds three layers of muscles. Superficial ones such as the bulbospongiosus control our external genitalia, allowing us to get aroused and have orgasms. A little farther into the body is the urogenital triangle, with muscles that encircle the urethra and vagina and strengthen the final and deepest layer, called the pelvic diaphragm, or floor. Made up of a group of muscles collectively called the levator ani, the pelvic floor, as its name suggests, is the main support for all of your pelvic organs—bladder, colon, uterus—holding them up from beneath.

Your pelvic floor is inherently strong and engaged, unconsciously controlled by your nervous system. Without these muscles actively working, your organs would fall out from between your legs. You'd be incontinent. In birth, these muscles play a critical role, wrapping around and supporting the baby's head as it makes its way out. (This is also why some women poop while bearing down and pushing during labor. The levator ani controls both functions.)

Surrounding all these bones, muscles, and organs are ligaments that attach muscle to bone, as well as several sheets of fascia, connective tissue layers that wrap around everything. Fasciae provide stability, holding organs in optimal functioning position. They also form the landscape for an extensive network of blood vessels, lymphatic vessels, and nerves, which give the whole region life and feeling.

In the long, messy, fluid- and excrement-soaked work of childbirth, the muscles of our pelvic floor can take a massive beating. It's believed that one in three mothers sustain pelvic floor injuries while giving birth.[1] During delivery, the skin around the vagina and the perineum, the small sling of skin between the vagina and anus, has to stretch—or, more accurately, streeeeeeeeeeetch. This can lead to tearing, which sounds scary but is common and easily repaired with stitches. Beneath the skin, the muscles also stretch—up to three times their usual length!—which may also lead to tearing and pulling. (No other human muscle can stretch even twice its length without tearing, so let's just acknowledge once and for all that what the female body is capable of is nothing short of heroic.)

During a Cesarean section, an incision is made in your lower abdomen and multiple layers of your body are cut through and/or moved out of the way: skin, fat, fascia, abdominal muscles (they are pulled apart and pushed to the sides); the peritoneum (a thin layer that lines the abdominal cavity); the bladder, which sits on top of the lower uterus and is typically pulled out of the way by a metal retractor tool called, horrifyingly, the bladder blade; another layer of peritoneum; and, finally, the uterus itself.

After delivery, all of that stuff has to go back inside your body and get placed in the proper spots. The uterus is sutured and, along with the bladder, returned to its usual position. The peritoneum layers are left to heal themselves; the muscles and fats are pushed back into place by sterile, gloved hands. The thick fascia, which is the most important supporting layer of the abdomen, is repaired with more durable stitches. And, of course, the skin is sewn together with stitches designed to dissolve into a smooth scar over time.

Cesarean sections carry the same risks as any major surgery, including increased bleeding, reactions to anesthesia, blood clots, and various surgical injuries. Doctors are required by law to warn women about what could happen to their bodies during a Cesarean section, even though the details of what exactly they are cutting through are often left unsaid. No such warnings exist for vaginal birth, though they should: the risks of injury and damage are just as significant, and women should be prepared for them or, at the very least, be made aware of the possibilities.

No matter how you give birth, it requires all sorts of

stretching, pushing, squeezing, stitching, rearranging, resettling, and healing. As with most things in life, it doesn't always go smoothly.

Birth is physically grueling, a test of endurance often compared to running a marathon (though typically lasting many hours more). Naturally, there will always be physical consequences and possible injuries. But unlike the marathoner who trains for months and has plentiful resources—entire magazines and websites filled with the newest information on how best to prepare as well as how to recover from a grueling race—women are rarely given any instruction on how to heal after birth. And yet, there are simple things we can do to get our strength back, things that should be as common to us as doing calf stretches or using a foam roller. Preparing for childbirth without ever hearing about your levator ani muscle and pudendal nerve is like training for a marathon without hearing about your hamstrings or IT band.

In the immediate recovery period, new mothers are looking at a fair amount of discomfort, possibly pain, in their vaginas, vulvas, perinea, lower abdomens, backs, and hips. They're also likely looking at a flaming case of hemorrhoids. All of this superficial damage is normal and is often resolved with a bit of care, rest, and time.

New mothers are also at risk for diastasis recti, a condition in which the rectus abdominis muscles (commonly known as your abs), which are stretched during pregnancy and manually rearranged during a C-section, separate vertically along your midline. It's basically like having your six-pack divide into two separate three-packs. Diastasis recti is a common condition that affects between 30 and 70 percent of women in late pregnancy, and up to 60 percent of postpartum women.[2] Depending on the size of the separation (the gap can be several inches wide), diastasis recti can be both physically uncomfortable and embarrassing, and also threaten the stability of the organs beneath the abs.

Deep muscular and fascia tears, as well as nerve damage and scarring, can have long-term effects that take much longer to resolve and may require medical attention.

When it's in optimal condition, the pelvic floor, like the floor of your house, is straight and flat. But, after childbirth, it might be sloped. If the floor in your apartment is crooked, you can still live with it, but furniture may start to slide around a bit. The same is true for your body and organs.

When muscles are weakened and loosened, they are less taut and supportive. Fascia, which wraps around the organs and is embedded in their walls, can be stretched, torn, and damaged in both vaginal and C-section deliveries, which can mean organs moving around, slipping into places they shouldn't be. This condition is called prolapse and it might manifest a few weeks, years, or even decades after you give birth. It can sometimes require surgery to repair.

C-section scarring, though it is only visible on the surface of the skin, actually happens at multiple levels. While the incision is delicate and an immediate source of pain when it comes to moving, lifting, stretching, and changing positions (all of which are required when caring for a newborn), the superficial discomfort eventually fades. Inside the body, though, scar tissue forms in the fascia and uterus—and it's not the same texture or composition as the surrounding tissue. Scars, both internal and external, can pull and push on surrounding tissues and organs, creating tension, pressure, and tightness. Scar tissue can also push on the pudendal nerve, the main nerve that serves the pelvic area, which itself can be stretched and injured during birth, scrambling or sending unpleasant sensations throughout your pelvis.

Prolapse and other pelvic floor disorders carry a range of symptoms, as individual as each person who gives birth. You might feel pain during sex, or less sexual sensation. It might hurt to exercise, and exercise and movement could cause you to pee your pants. Incontinence, both urinary and fecal, could occur not only when you're running or jumping but when you sneeze or laugh.

After my first pelvic floor strengthening class, I immediately called a close friend who is a fitness instructor and personal trainer. Did she know about the peeing thing?

"Oh yeah," she told me. "I can always tell who the women who have given birth in my group classes are. They're the ones in the back, afraid to jump up and down."

The majority of women who give birth experience some sort of tearing in their pelvic skin and muscles. Again, it is common and normal. But for more than 10 percent of women, the tearing is enough to lead to incontinence.[3] One-third of women suffer from a pelvic floor disorder, which includes prolapse and urinary and fecal incontinence.[4] Eighty percent of those women are mothers—our mothers, sisters, aunts, cousins, coworkers, and friends.

My friend Rivka experienced slight tearing of her perineum

after the birth of her first child. She was stitched up and, after about two months of tenderness and mild pain, healed. She didn't have any tearing with the birth of her second child two years later, but she developed a rectocele, a condition in which the rectum collapses and presses into the back wall of the vagina. It's the result of damage done to the rectovaginal fascia while pushing.

Rivka could actually see the spot where it was happening; it appeared as a pink bulge when she looked at her vagina with a hand mirror (or, to be more accurate, when her midwife insisted that she, reluctant, look at her vagina at her postpartum appointment). She described the sensations of the rectocele as being as unsettling as having to look at her bulge that first time. She was haunted by feelings of heaviness and pressure, as though something might fall out of her at any time.

"It wasn't exactly pain, and I didn't have to poop or pee all the time, but it just wasn't right," she said. "I spent a lot of time worrying, is something coming out of my vagina? I'd put my finger in to check but there was nothing there."

The discomfort was at its worst when she was very active, walking long distances, or spending a day on her feet. Or, just as often, performing the daily activities of taking care of two young children.

It affected her sex life, too. The first time Rivka's husband went down on her after having her second baby, she stopped him to ask nervously, "Can you feel it?" He couldn't—and anyway, he didn't care, so he carried on. But she said it was embarrassing to have to ask, even if it wasn't a big deal to him.

"I feel really lucky that my midwives were so wonderful,"

she said of the care she received. "They told me it was normal, that I needed to keep an eye on it. That I still had pelvic tone and that I could improve the situation by doing Kegels."

Even with that initial encouragement and care, though, it took a full year for her vagina to feel normal again.

"And honestly," Rivka said matter-of-factly, "it's never going to be the same."

I did not expect to have a C-section, but the next day—groggy, in pain, swollen—I was forced to adjust to my new reality. I was encouraged to get up and walk. So in the late afternoon, I mustered the strength to shakily walk to the bathroom and wash my face. I looked down at my body, which had been pumped full of fluids for a full day, and saw that the bandages over my incision were bulging. As I leaned over the sink, the dressing popped open, spewing a bloody liquid that landed on the bathroom floor with a dramatic and terrifying *splat!* I looked at my puffy face in the mirror, bags under my eyes, tears streaming down my cheeks, and thought, *This is my life now.*

I expected my postpartum body to be tired. To feel soft, weak, leaky, oozy. I wasn't in any rush to "get my body back," mainly because I could barely make sense of the body I now had. I finally went for my first real walk a month after giving birth, and mostly out of necessity. For my baby, the "witching hour" was a very real thing—she would scream inconsolably between five and seven p.m. unless strapped inside a baby carrier and out walking the brisk fall streets.

I was prepared for the fact that a tender wound would dominate my lower abdomen for months. But here is what I was not prepared for: that after it healed, I would experience an entirely new pain. A pain in my hips—a constant, white-hot burning and tightening in the seam where my thighs met my crotch. It bothered me as I sat at my desk at work, as I stood at my desk at work, as I balanced on an exercise ball at my desk at work. It bothered me when I sat down to nurse, when I lay down in bed every night.

I couldn't fall asleep at night without "butterflying" my legs—lying on my back, bringing my legs up and the bottoms of my feet together like butterfly wings, and beating them for a few minutes. I am sure it irritated my husband, desperately trying to fall asleep next to me, trying to squeeze in rest before our infant eventually woke us with her screaming—but he was kind enough never to say anything. I rolled my hips on tennis balls, on purple yoga tune-up balls. I rolled on a foam roller. I scoured my anatomy book and thought perhaps the pain was related to tight psoas muscles and went to see a massage therapist. Afterward, she told me that while she had no doubt that I was experiencing pain, the problem was not muscular.

*

Pelvic pain and pelvic floor disorders are common after child-birth, but they are not normal. No one should have to live with this pain, nor the embarrassment, loneliness, and shame that often accompanies it. But even if a woman seeks help for her problems, she may not get the treatment she needs. A survey published in 2016 revealed that the majority of primary care physicians didn't screen for prolapse and that 50 percent believe that the condition is rare.[5] (Meanwhile, studies show that prolapse may affect over half of all women and that some degree of prolapse is extremely common in older women.)[6]

The physical and psychological discomfort that women express—if they feel comfortable enough expressing it to their doctors—is often met with an answer similar to, "Well, you just had a baby." It's as though we are not allowed—let alone entitled—to expect more. To expect health.

In cultures throughout the world—Asian, Latin American, and African—tradition dictates that mothers be confined to the home for up to forty days after giving birth. They are tended to by their mothers, mothers-in-law, and other female community members who cook and clean the house for them, who hold and tend to the baby, as well as show them how to care for and feed their infants.

The over two-thousand-year-old Chinese tradition of *zuo yue zi* ("sitting the month") is rooted in the belief that a woman who has given birth has lost blood, heat, and yang, and is therefore susceptible to cold, or yin. She is given only hot liquids and fed medicinal stews—fish soup with goji berries and dates, pigs' feet with peanuts—to restore energy and warmth. She is prohibited from drinking cold water, going outside, and exposing herself to cold air—even bathing. While the many women who still follow *zuo yue zi* today no longer follow the strictest rules and choose to take showers and baths, the ritual is the same: to rest and replenish their "broken bodies."

In colonial America, it was common practice for women to

"lie in" for three to four weeks following birth. But obviously, that tradition has faded. Today, when many women live far away from extended family, we have few rituals or traditions to support women as they move through the biggest transition of their lives. In other countries, as well as in some tight-knit immigrant communities, there is a more robust support system of female relatives and community members who tend to new mothers.

Additionally, there is pressure for new moms to get back out there instead of "lying in." In modern America, a woman at rest is often a woman effectively removed from the world—not working, not earning money, and falling behind. We've managed to turn a necessity of life into a liability.

If a woman's concerns are dismissed (or never even asked about) at her first postpartum appointment, she's probably less likely to raise the issue again. But when would she raise it? In the United States, the standard of care is one postpartum checkup six weeks after you give birth. That's it. New babies get a one-week, two-month, four-month, six-month, nine-month, and one-year wellness visit. In countries throughout Europe, midwives make home visits to see how new babies—and mothers—are faring. But after six weeks, American mothers are on their own.

It doesn't have to be this way.

April Bolding, a Seattle-based physical therapist who specializes in treating women's health issues, has worked with new mothers for more than twenty years. When I asked her what could be done to better meet the needs of postpartum women, she said, "We should have routine physical therapy for the pelvic floor starting at six weeks post birth. There is no reason why we can't do this."

Bolding—who also works as a childbirth educator and a doula—said that in her experience, postpartum women are an underserved population when it comes to treatment and rehabilitation for pregnancy- and birth-related injuries. It was because of this that she decided to focus her practice solely on women's health issues, specifically the pelvic floor.

Physical therapy can be a powerful intervention for all new mothers, even if they are not experiencing major problems. "Birth involves muscles," she said, "and physical therapy concerns muscles, alignment, and activity."

In one consultation, therapists can assess the strength, muscle, tone, and tension of the pelvic floor and recommend exercises unique to each woman. Women with diastasis recti can be taught how to engage their transverse abdominals and pelvic floor, which is crucial to recovery. Women are often told to do Kegel exercises before and after birth, but that is just one repetitive motion. A single motion cannot solve a range of issues affecting a variety of muscles. There is no magical, one-size-fits-all solution to our pelvic problems.

Prolapse varies in severity and is graded on a scale of 1 to 3 (3 being the most severe). A person could have grade 2 bladder prolapse, where the bladder sags into the vagina, caused by damage to the fascia that supports the organ. While therapeutic exercises cannot repair the fascia itself, they can strengthen the muscle tone around the vagina, which in turn can support and push the bladder into a better position, closer to grade 1, making it less disruptive and less uncomfortable.

These types of interventions are not only helpful for women who have given birth vaginally but also for women who have undergone C-sections. After the incision has healed, a therapist can mobilize and massage both the internal and external scar tissue. (If you don't have access to therapy, there are quite a few YouTube videos that show you how to massage your scar.) The more scar tissue is moved, the softer it becomes, and the less havoc it may wreak on your bladder, bowels, sex life, and lower back.

Some pelvic floor problems require the attention of a urogynecologist. A urogynecologist could fit women for a pessary, a sort of custom-made bra for the internal organs that can be inserted and used to help lift and support them. And, if necessary, surgery can be used to repair problems.

Internal organ bras might raise eyebrows in the United States, but in countries like France, where every woman who gives birth is referred for *la rééducation périnéale*, individual treatment to strengthen a new mother's pelvic floor, no one bats an eye. This perineal reeducation, which is subsidized by the government, might also include biofeedback therapy, in which a small joystick/dildo with electrodes is inserted into the vagina and one plays video games with it as it measures the strength of muscle contractions. This is everyday life for new French mothers, whose government views physical therapy as a long-term investment in their health.

It begs the question: Why can't we offer similar types of support and benefits to new mothers in the United States? The technology is available and there are a growing number of providers who specialize in pelvic floor therapy (they help meet the growing demand of mothers actively seeking help). But none of this is widely known, discussed, or promoted, even though some insurance policies cover rehabilitation. Just one postpartum appointment focused on the pelvis could save money and time for both mothers and physicians down the road. Armed with a few personally prescribed exercises, women could begin dealing with problems that, left unaddressed, could lead to incontinence, chronic back pain, and other conditions that will eventually require treatment. It also, importantly, sends a message to new mothers that their postpartum injuries are not imagined or trivial—that they, and their bodies, are deserving of care and attention.

You probably know someone who has torn their ACL (anterior cruciate ligament), a knee injury that is common to sports like basketball and soccer. For the majority of people who want to maintain full range of motion, an ACL injury is repaired by arthroscopic surgery, a modern, minimally invasive method developed to reduce pain, complications, and recovery time. As part of their ACL recovery, patients are put on a program of physical therapy that includes multiple phases of exercises that can last up to six months. This is the standard care that the roughly two hundred thousand people who experience an ACL injury each year receive. There is no such standard protocol for the treatment of pelvic floor disorders, which affect up to 1.3 million of the 4 million American women who give birth annually.

The majority of ACL tears in this country occurs in men. I have a hard time believing that the discrepancy in attention and care is coincidental.

Without women bearing children, our species ceases to exist. How can we not place a premium on the care of the mother? We deserve better.

*

My husband, daughter, and I all see the same family physician. Our doctor cared for me after my miscarriage, he advised my husband on how to deal with the two-inch-long splinter he once got in his hand while dusting the house, and he delivered our daughter. When she was a baby, he treated both of us. At her one-week appointment, he took the time to look at my incision, replacing the dressing with little butterfly bandages. At her subsequent appointments, he checked to see that it was healing properly and asked me how I was doing. At her one-year checkup, I asked him about the pain in my hips and if it could be related to pregnancy and childbirth, as I was certain it was.

"Maybe," he replied, adding that a lot of people had tight hip joints. He suggested stretching. He wasn't dismissive, but that was the end of the discussion; our twenty-minute appointment was over.

Little did he know that I was already doing pigeon pose every morning and every evening. That every day for weeks I had been lying on my dining-room table, my spine lined up with one of its outer edges, dangling half of my body off it, because that was one of the only ways to achieve the stretch that my hips were demanding.

I left the clinic convinced that I was going to be living with chronic hip pain for the rest of my life. And I found myself thinking the same thing so many other women are made to wonder: *What did you expect? You had a baby.*

Remembering the pale, oozing, hospital gown–clad woman I had seen in the hospital mirror months before, I thought: *This is who I am now. A broken person who no one knows how to fix.*

For weeks, which turned into months, I continued my daily routine of lying on the floor (and dining-room table), stretching and rolling. It became a ritual of movement and stillness, deep breaths taken to cut through pain, fear, and frustration. Somewhere, slowly, within that stillness, I discovered that I wanted to understand my body better, to be in tune with it. To heal it.

As I lay there, my husband usually nearby reading ESPN .com on his phone or watching television, the baby would cry from her crib. Just as I would start to get up, he would stop me and say, "Stay there, I got this." Eventually, I stopped getting up. The more I allowed myself to stay still, the more I realized how important it was for me to care for myself, my body, the one that increasingly seemed to exist only for other people's survival and happiness.

Along with stretching, I started moving—and dancing. I took ballet classes as a kid, performed in musicals in high school, and, in my twenties, took a few hip-hop classes. Somewhere along the way, though, I stopped doing it except in my living room, at wedding receptions, or during the occasional night out. But almost immediately after my daughter started walking, just before she turned one, she started dancing, too. She had a rhythm inside her that she needed to follow. (We all do, we just get better at ignoring it as we get older.) We merged our interests into nightly living-room dance parties. Aside from the classical music that came out of her Little Einstein "radio," the first song she really got down to was Ariana Grande's "Into You."

One night at a friend's dinner party, as my daughter and I danced to Taylor Swift's "Shake It Off," another friend mentioned that the next morning he was going to a movement class called Dance Church. It was taught by a professional dancer but open to anyone—a guided improvisational class set to pop music. The next morning, I went. It was part aerobics class, part free-form movement, no mirrors in the studio, no rules.

When, at one point, we were instructed to "grind your crotch down into the floor" during a Drake song, someone near me giggled uncomfortably. I realized that this was the easiest, most liberating thing my vagina had been asked to do all year, so I threw my head back, grinned, and humped the floor. Over the next few weeks, I was surprised to discover that a good chunk of the movements we did in class were geared toward the hips—the most problematic area of my body.

"*Open up your underwear line,*" the instructor said. I followed directions dutifully. As I moved the seams where my thighs meet my crotch, they creaked like wooden doors on old brass hinges.

"*Get it juicy.*" I made a circle with my hips and looked over my shoulder to see that suddenly my ass had morphed into the ripe, round peach emoji.

"*Spread your crack.*" I wasn't entirely sure how to do this, so I closed my eyes and swirled my peach emoji ass around as though its cheeks might touch opposite walls of the studio.

Aside from sex and childbirth, when are you ever told to open up this part of yourself? In everyday life, it might be embarrassing, but, in the context of Missy Elliott, it's necessary.

The more I moved, the more the pain went away. I started going to class every week, sometimes twice. My husband, happy to see me no longer uncomfortable, set aside the hours each week to be at home with our daughter so I could go. While no physician ever gave me a diagnosis for my pain, my body told me everything I needed to know. I was moving the parts of my body that were being pushed and pulled, tightened and tensed. But it was more than therapeutic—it was freeing. In class, I didn't care what anyone thought of my body. I was too busy having fun to notice.

The pain in my hips wasn't completely gone. It took over two years after giving birth for it to fade. But even now, if I don't move regularly, the discomfort comes roaring back. I think about how my friend's vagina didn't arrive at its "new normal" until a full year later. It is easy for mothers to focus our attention away from our own needs and onto those of our tiny, helpless babies—after all, they will only be this young once.

But we will never be this young again, either.

Healing—and acceptance of our shifting forms—can happen sooner, or at least with less mental anguish, if we told women the facts about their bodies and what happens to it in childbirth. That it wrecks you. But that the wreckage is something we are necessarily meant to withstand and survive.

Perhaps health-care providers don't tell us the truth because they are afraid of scaring us. And yet, the potential damage we could do to our babies in utero—by eating seafood, drinking a glass of wine, cleaning the house, relaxing in a hot tub—is lorded over us for nine months. Afterward, when pregnancy is over, the medical establishment essentially tells us we're on our own to figure everything out.

Maybe the reason we don't tell women about the ways their bodies will change after they give birth is because, quite simply, health-care providers don't know. They've been trained to prioritize the health of newborn babies but not newly born mothers.

Or maybe it's something worse that skews our priorities: that we don't want women to be connected to themselves, empowered, asking questions, demanding action. Because being in touch with our pelvic region puts us in touch with that which is the most powerful—and pleasurable.

The full anatomy of the clitoris—the female sex organ that everyone on earth has lived in close proximity to while in their mother's bodies—wasn't fully known until 1998, when an Australian urologist named Helen O'Connell published her groundbreaking findings. *Just two decades ago, we had no clue what the clitoris was.* Until O'Connell came along, modern anatomy texts had presented the clitoris "as minute or not represented at all."[7] Through extensive dissection and, later, magnetic resonance imaging (MRI), O'Connell defined the true size and shape of the clitoris, which has ten times more tissue than any anatomy textbook or picture at the doctor's office shows.

Along with the glans of the clitoris, the only external part of the organ, there are the crura, two legs that are each up to ten centimeters long. They extend downward, surrounding the vagina on either side. Vestibular bulbs also flank the vagina; they are bundles of erectile tissue that, during arousal, swell and stimulate the area. The clitoris isn't a wee thing hovering above the vagina; it's actually a dynamic entity that holds it in a devoted embrace. It holds eight thousand nerve endings—twice the amount of the penis. It is the only organ in the human body built solely for pleasure.

There is so much more to the female body than we realize.

If you are, rightfully, a little nervous about what might happen in childbirth, you should know that your body shifts and changes, readying itself as best it can. If you were to feel your vagina and cervix throughout pregnancy, you would find that, when they are close to giving birth, they feel completely different.

"At term," said April Bolding, "the tissues are so much more buttery and extensible."

It is okay to touch yourself, to know yourself in this way. In fact, it may help you approach birth—and everything else that follows—with less fear, more strength.

*

Since she was a baby, my daughter has shown an instinctual curiosity about her body. During diaper changes, she would reach down, her little fingers exploring the area of her crotch. She would find her clitoris, hidden under the fleshy hood where her tiny labia meet, then rub, poke, and tickle it. It made her laugh.

We encouraged her to touch herself and told her what these parts of her body were called: *clitoris, vulva, vagina*. We asked her what she was doing.

"I touch my va-nina," she replied.

And how does it feel?

"Like corn," she answered, her eyes twinkling, and with a knowing smile that seemed to convey the sweetness of it. Corn!

She calls her arm her arm, her neck her neck, her hair her hair, and so she will call her vagina her vagina. It is what it is, after all, and it is all hers. We will give her parts names so that she can tell us when these things feel good, when they hurt. So we can teach her how to keep them healthy and clean.

I want my daughter always to know that her parts are hers alone. That right now we help her with them but ultimately they are for her to do with as she pleases. And that one day, when and only if she wants, she can let someone else touch her there, too.

I have no idea who she will become. But eventually her body will be ready to menstruate. Maybe one day she will have a child of her own. I don't want the workings of her body to ever be a mystery to her, something that she doesn't understand or looks to others for it to feel complete. I don't want her to be well into adulthood before she knows how she likes to be touched, and how to ask someone for that. Becoming a mother may be one of our most culturally traditional acts, but it is also the place where we can break with our most limiting, oppressive traditions.

We dance in the living room nearly every night. To her favorite Drake song, which she has renamed "Hot Dog Bling." It keeps my body happy. It makes her body, which she is just learning about, happy. The high ceilings of our house echo with our squeals and shouts.

She gets down on all fours, she shakes her head, she does "down dog" and lifts her right leg high. She plays air guitar, although it looks more like a karate chop or someone manically moving a violin bow through the air.

I lift my leg, Mama.
This my booty, I shake my booty.

I shake my booty, too. I watch her and think how self-discovery is the bravest, most rewarding act, one that goes on for a lifetime.

CHAPTER 10

UNFOLDING

I woke up one morning, after an automatic software update that happened while I slept, to discover that my iPhone had changed into a machine that could now recognize the faces in my photos and sort them into albums. My phone contained more than four hundred pictures of my daughter: there she was, spread out through seven albums, each one collected under a different thumbnail image of her face. Because I live with her every day, changes in her features—her chubby cheeks shedding their roundness, the lightening of her brown hair—happen almost imperceptibly, until suddenly one day I look at her and realize she is not the baby or little girl she once was.

If I knew anything about facial recognition technology, I'm sure I would have found this disturbing. But mostly I felt grateful to my phone for the perspective, for allowing me to see my girl, clearly, at so many different stages during her brief time on earth.

What struck me as odd, though, was that my devices

recognized me as two different people and, accordingly, divided me into two albums. I scrolled through both of them, trying to detect what could account for the split. I immediately looked to see if the photos were grouped chronologically; they were not. After several scroll-throughs, I still couldn't figure it out. Had I lost or gained weight? Was it that regrettable haircut I had gotten? A few days later, I realized what the difference was. It was embarrassingly obvious: in some of the pictures I am wearing my glasses, in the others, contact lenses.

In that moment, though, I understood that all the while I was scouring those photos, what I had really been looking for was reassurance, for proof of something I already knew: becoming a mother had changed me.

I'm not talking about the superficial changes like the smooth, raised scar on my lower abdomen, or the strong left arm that allows me to carry thirty-plus pounds of child on my hip as I stir soup on the stove, or my breasts that, empty of the milk with which they were once so often swollen, now seem to inch their way toward the ground with every passing day. No, having a baby changed me in a way that I felt deep down—in my blood, bones, and cells—somewhere inside me that I couldn't quite place.

I am not the person I once was.

*

In Greek mythology, the chimera is a fire-breathing beast that is part lion, part snake, and part goat. In the natural world, the chimera lends its name to describe organisms such as coral and slime mold, single beings that are actually composed of two living things. In medicine, microchimerism refers to a body's harboring of cells or DNA that are genetically distinct from itself—genetic material that developed in the body of another person. Because the foreign cells were believed to be present in only small amounts, the prefix "micro" is used.

While the idea of another person's cells living in your body may sound like the creepy, far-fetched stuff of science fiction, microchimerism—once thought to be a rare, novel occurrence—is actually an everyday reality for mothers and, perhaps, all humans.

Emerging science reveals that most likely all of us have at least a few cells from our mothers—and, astonishingly, other people including maternal grandmothers, and possibly older siblings—in our bodies.[1] Throughout pregnancy, our cells commingle, crossing borders—the placenta, the blood-brain barrier—that were once thought to be impenetrable. Mothers' cells take up residency in the fetuses growing inside them and, when these babies emerge into the world, they often do so armed with some of their mothers' cells. These microchimeric cells are not merely passive travelers; some grow, thrive, and persist in our bodies for decades, lifetimes, and even generations.

In 1996, Dr. Diana Bianchi, a geneticist at Tufts University in Boston, found male DNA in the blood of women decades after they had given birth—twenty-seven years in one case.[2] The women were in good health, so, aside from being present in these mothers' bodies, what exactly these fetal cells were up to was unknown. Further research revealed that the microchimeric cells are able to survive for so long because they are stem or stem-related cells, capable of dividing indefinitely and developing into a wide range of specialized cells, including beating heart muscle or rapidly firing neurons.

A decade and a half later, scientists at the University of Alberta looked for fetal microchimerism in the brains of fifty-nine women following their deaths. Each of these women had given birth to a son. The scientists detected male DNA in 63 percent of the women's brains and in multiple regions throughout them. The oldest subject was ninety-four years old, meaning her son's cells had lived in her body for most of her life.[3] Our children are, quite literally, frequent and widespread residents of our brains.

After decades of research, we are just now beginning to understand the impact that microchimeric cells have on our health and bodies, and even our sense of self.

"A whopping 6-plus percent of DNA [in a mother's blood] in the third trimester can be fetal," said Dr. J. Lee Nelson, a rheumatologist at the Fred Hutchinson Cancer Research Center in Seattle. "That's amazing, and not actually *micro* at all."

"So if you felt weird during late pregnancy," she laughed, "you had a good reason to feel weird."

In the final weeks of my pregnancy, I was beyond uncomfortable: it was as though I had outgrown my own skin and, occasionally, I felt the urge to crawl out of it entirely. Maybe, I thought as I listened to Nelson, what I was feeling were parts of my daughter hitching a ride through my blood vessels, doing recon, looking for an exit.

Nelson has been studying the exchange of fetal and maternal cells, as well as what roles these cells might play in our bodies, for over three decades. She began her work studying autoimmune diseases, but during a research fellowship in the 1980s, a pregnant patient changed the course of her entire career.

"[The patient] had very severe rheumatoid arthritis that went into complete remission while she was pregnant," recalled Nelson. "And then as soon as she delivered—boom—it was back. I thought, 'Now this is something worthwhile, something worth studying.'"

After a pause, she added, "I was actually quite surprised to see there was very little research done on it." It's a familiar sentiment, one shared by all of the scientists and health-care workers I interviewed for this book: immediately after recognizing an aspect of women's health as rich territory for inquiry, they discovered that there was a dearth of existing research or funds allocated to research that topic.

Autoimmune diseases, which include such disorders as rheumatoid arthritis, multiple sclerosis, and lupus, are diseases that are caused, in part, by the body's immune system attacking its own healthy cells. These diseases disproportionately affect women, who make up 80 percent of all known cases of autoimmune disease in the United States. When Nelson began her work in this area, the prevailing—and limited—thinking behind the gender discrepancy was, in her words, "hormones, hormones, hormones." (Hormones, in fairness, do play a complex role in the body, acting as chemical messengers that affect cognitive function, the cardiovascular system, and various other systems. They are responsible for more than just our reproductive health.)

But Nelson believed that explanation to be inadequate. She knew that women are less affected by these disorders in their twenties and thirties—the traditional childbearing years when hormone levels are higher and fluctuations happen regularly as part of the monthly menstrual cycle—than in their forties, fifties, and sixties. She wondered if the fetal cells that interacted with a woman's body during pregnancy might play a role in the development of autoimmune issues decades later.

"It seemed to me pretty self-evident that if you've got an autoimmune disease, you should look at what's immunologic," she said. "And with pregnancy, the fact is that a woman is somehow managing to carry—to tolerate—a half-foreign being."

Starting with a small grant, Nelson began testing her hypothesis that fetal cells impact a mother's long-term health. She partnered with Dr. Diana Bianchi, the geneticist who discovered the microchimeric cells that persisted in healthy mothers after childbirth. Working together, they found that women with the autoimmune disease scleroderma—a debilitating chronic illness in which a person's skin and connective tissue harden and tighten—had higher levels of fetal microchimerism than healthy women. Fetal cells have since been linked to other maternal illnesses including multiple sclerosis and preeclampsia.

"In the beginning, the knee-jerk response to microchimerism is 'Yikes, these aren't my cells, they must all be bad players,'" said Nelson. "But that wasn't my assumption because I knew that these cells also exist in normal, healthy people."

And indeed, the impact of these cells isn't always negative. If a mother has undergone surgery to have her baby, for example, the cells may help her heal. Fetal cells have been found in Cesarean section scars, as well as other healed wounds, suggesting they play a role in maternal injury recovery. Microchimeric cells have also been found throughout women's bodies in healthy organs such as the breasts, heart, thyroid, lungs, liver, and, as mentioned previously, the brain. Some research indicates that these cells may even play a role in disease prevention.

Why would these foreign cells want to preserve the health of their host body? It makes perfect sense when you think about it: a healthy mother is better able to provide for the needs of her baby. There is a biological imperative to the function of microchimeric cells. Fetal cells have been found in breast tissue and breast milk, hinting that they could have a hand in increasing their own food supply.

The complicated relationship that parents and their children have out in the "real world"—by turns exhausting, exhilarating, soul-crushing, and life-affirming, played out against a tableau of sleep deprivation, tears, and emotions—actually begins silently, deep within the uterus, with the invisible swapping of cells and genetic material. It mirrors the early, contradictory scientific findings about microchimerism. The daily relationship between parents and children are inherently contradictory; it's push-pull, hurt feelings and reconciliation, a constant negotiation over independence and freedom. We need each other as much as we want to be free of each other. Children have both positive and negative effects on their parents; we are engaged in what researchers at Arizona State University call "evolutionary cooperation and conflict."

For the last few years, Lee Nelson has devoted much of her time to studying the impact of microchimerism on cancer. Pregnancy is known to have a long-term effect of reducing the risk of breast cancer.[4] While we don't yet know if there is a direct relationship between microchimerism and breast cancer, we do know that mothers without the disease have higher amounts of microchimeric cells in their bodies. And for the last few years, Nelson has also been looking at what she calls "mother as anti-cancer drug": early results from her studies suggest that maternal microchimerism—cells from the mother present in fetal umbilical cord blood—are effective against the development of acute leukemia.[5]

Perhaps most significantly, what Nelson and her colleagues have proven over the last thirty years is that the perceived novelty of microchimerism, like the creature it derives its name from, is a myth, an illusion. It's actually commonplace.

If the human body's proclivity to hold on to others' cells is so fundamental to our nature—inherent in the process of reproduction—why do we know so little about it?

After completing her study of microchimerism and scleroderma in the late 1990s, Nelson submitted her findings to a leading medical journal.

"I got back a nice personal letter saying, 'Why don't you do this in mice instead?'" she said. Nelson's study was eventually published in another journal, but the letter—which she still has—is emblematic of the ongoing struggle for legitimacy when it comes to the study of female reproductive health.

For years, Nelson used data from organ transplant studies. While transplants can sometimes lead to chimerism, it occurs frequently and naturally in pregnancy. Pregnancy is far more common than organ transplant surgery, and yet when Nelson began working there was virtually no information available about the chimerism it produces.

"It seems a little crazy that I should have to borrow a lot of my information from transplanters," said Nelson. "There is a whole lot more information [in pregnancy] that we could try to understand and learn from. It really should be center stage."

Diana Bianchi, the Tufts University geneticist who was one of Nelson's first collaborators, is now the director of the Eunice Kennedy Shriver National Institute of Child Health and Human Development (NICHD), the federal government agency that funds research into fertility, pregnancy, growth, and development. The institute's mission is to study the vital, complex process of human development from the beginning of life until death.

In 2016, Congress granted the NICHD a total of $1.3 billion to do its work. Its peer, the National Cancer Institute, received four times that amount of money, or $5.2 billion. The National Institute of Allergy and Infectious Diseases received $4.6 billion, and the National Heart, Lung, and Blood Institute, $3.1 billion.[6]

Microchimerism is an emerging field of science, and more studies are needed to fully understand its impact on human health. But while these fetal and maternal cells are only now finding their way into mainstream scientific study and public consciousness, it's likely that they have existed within mothers for tens of millions of years. They are, in the words of Arizona State University biologist and researcher Dr. Melissa Wilson Sayres, "something that humans have been evolving with since before we were humans."[7]

We have known for some time that the long-term health of mothers and their children is impacted by the physical journey of pregnancy. We now also know that the long-term health of mothers and their children is impacted by the physical journey that takes place after pregnancy. We owe it to women, and our children, to dedicate the necessary resources to better understanding this emerging but potentially life-changing science.

*

A few weeks after my daughter was born, my husband went back to work. My friend Abbie, who had given birth a few months before I did, came over one day, bringing her baby and lunch for us both. Abbie was my main source of new mom information. She was the person I texted questions about nipples and diaper rash to at eleven p.m. or five a.m., and she almost always answered immediately. I remember visiting her in the days following her son's birth, bearing a pork shoulder braised with apple cider and onions. Five months pregnant and curious about her journey, I sat with her on her couch and asked her how she was doing.

Abbie looked at me, tears welling in her eyes, and spoke with a clarity that shook me and will stay with me forever: "For the most part, I'm fine. I'm happy. But every day around five, I get overwhelmed. It's hard. It feels like I am falling in love and getting my heart broken at the same time."

When Abbie came over that day, I confessed to her the heavy secret I had been carrying around in my bones for weeks: I was pretty sure I was a totally different person (kind of). She looked at me and nodded. "Yes," she said simply, "I'm not the same person I was. Something inside me is different."

I was relieved. I was not alone. For the moment, it was enough.

The scientists at Arizona State write that studying microchimerism has "potentially important implications for our understanding of health and disease pathology, including lactation science, thyroid diseases, autoimmune diseases, cancer and even maternal emotional and psychological health postpartum."

As I read this paper, I was struck by the use of the word "even" in qualifying women's emotional and psychological health. I understood that it was likely used because we know the least about how fetal microchimerism may impact women's psychological health, but it was difficult not to read it as indicative of the fact that the emotional well-being and mental health of mothers is still very much an afterthought.

When it comes to motherhood, we tend to gloss over, ignore, judge, or, even worse, pathologize difficult emotions. Intentionally or not, we shame and isolate women who don't have the joyful pregnancy and postpartum experiences our culture expects rather than helping or really making an effort to understand them. The biological, psychological, and social underpinnings of maternal health are complex—and problems manifest in a highly individual manner. But we know that 80 percent of new mothers report a range of mood changes, and that as many as one in seven mothers will experience postpartum depression and/or anxiety.[8] That's over six hundred thousand women in the United States weathering illnesses that are natural, often uncontrollable, consequences of an essential, life-sustaining process. We should know much more about it than we do.

Motherhood requires weathering daily traumas (both big and small), learning to dwell in the mundane, and cultivating patience. To be a mother is to be on intimate, daily terms with conflict, sadness, joy, anger—all the big emotions, all of them urgent, right there under the skin ready to jump out. You can't live in the close proximity of an infant's cries, a toddler's frustration, a child's squeals, without some of that intensity affecting you.

Children are helpless; they show us our capacity for love. Fetal cells sometimes help us heal our wounds; sometimes they cause hurt we could never imagine. Mothers, in nurturing and giving to their child, are ripped apart and worn down but are also given a new dimension.

My daughter stopped breast-feeding just after she turned two. In the months leading up to it, she nursed just one or two times a day, maybe a little bit more when we spent all day together on the weekends. It wasn't for nourishment—at this point, she was putting down full meals—but for comfort:

when she wasn't feeling well or when, after a tantrum or crying fit, she needed a little emotional reset.

The process of weaning took a lot longer than I expected. I told myself that I was following her lead, but the truth is that I was also dragging my heels. She was becoming an increasingly mobile, squirmy, and active person. Nursing was the only time that she would let me hold her, uninterrupted, for five or ten minutes. As much as I wanted to be free of the way she took liberties with me, treating my body as if it were her own personal buffet or jungle gym, I would sniff her scalp and never want to let go.

One afternoon, after a particularly painful, loud, and tear-soaked standoff about one of the many things that adults regard as trivial but, to a toddler, is monumental, we reconciled over a bit of breast milk. As I nursed her, weary of her and her need for me, my gaze drifted up and out the window, my thoughts to everywhere else I could be, all the things I could be doing if I wasn't trapped here with her. Suddenly, my daughter's tiny hand reached up and directed my face back to hers. We stared at each other, studied each other. And just like that, she had restored order to my world, which she had single-handedly, violently shaken just moments before. I wished that I could summon a simple gesture to repair all the misunderstandings and hurt that have marked my relationship with my own mother over the years.

The reality of microchimerism requires us to reconsider our concept of "self" entirely. We are never alone; we never have been. With all of our interactions, we bring not just ourselves but how we were raised—the people who raised us, their values, virtues, and flaws—to the table. And it's likely that all of us hold cells from someone else inside us.

Microchimerism occurs in pregnancies that end in miscarriage or are terminated. Even if a pregnancy ends early, the cells of that fetus may live on. Even if a child dies, a bit of his life continues in his mother's body. Microchimerism is part of how life begins, and it is part of how life goes on.

The idea of being constituted by others goes against the myth of America's rugged individualism. Our culture prizes personal achievement and fulfillment, but places much less value on paying attention to and caring for the needs of others. Parenting requires that you put someone else's needs ahead of your own. We are made up of others, we are changed by others, and we need others. The obliteration of your old self can be disorienting and disheartening, but it can also be a source of great power and transformation.

Mothers understand this.

*

Female bodies were built to accommodate other bodies. Even after pregnancy, a mother's body continues to give, continues to change and develop. Birth tears you open, sometimes violently, and you don't just pull yourself back together and return to your previous state. Your organs have shifted, your muscles have torn, there are extra folds and layers to your skin and soul.

I have tried many times to come up with the proper metaphor so other people can understand this fundamental, though often imperceptible, change. What is it like?

What I've found, over and over, is that I have none. Until it happened to me, I'd never experienced anything like it. And, perhaps if the circumstances of my life were different, I might never have noticed or spent much time thinking about it. For many mothers, thinking about this requires precious minutes stolen for themselves amid work, family, child care, life. But it is real, whether or not we are able to acknowledge it.

We are still at a point where we lack stories—diverse stories—about pregnancy and motherhood. Only if we tell and hear these stories do we have a chance at understanding the experience, of making progress. Only if we see these stories as inherently valuable will we appreciate women as we should. Only then will we have the chance of creating a society that listens to, champions, and supports us for the marvelously strong and vulnerable beings that we are.

Everything that has happened since the egg that would be my daughter was fertilized—pregnancy, birth, returning to outside work, solid foods, crawling, walking, running, potty training, climbing—has only ever felt like a beginning. Just when I get used to some routine, some pattern, it changes. Beginning after beginning opens up in my life—reflection upon reflection in a room of mirrors, vault after vault of Romanesque arches.[9] It is more than I could have ever imagined.

And yet I wonder—sometimes fear—what will happen if I have another child, what that pregnancy will do to me. I have only recently begun to stop thinking of myself as two separate people, the former me and the mother, divided neatly into albums.

Recently, a friend on Facebook posted about her impending return to work after the birth of her son. She missed her practice as a therapist but was worried about what working would be like after what she called "the biggest shift in my life so far." Many women chimed in with comments of support and their own stories. The last time I saw this friend was over ten years ago, before she moved to another city, well before either of us was married, back when two a.m. belonged to us, the night, and last call, not the cries of our babies. But I felt compelled to add my voice to the chorus of well-wishers. I told her that, nearly three years after the birth of my daughter, I still haven't fully reconciled the pre- and post-baby parts of me.

"It's an unfolding!" she replied, giving me the word I had been searching for to explain what happened—what is still happening.

At first, I see the unfurling of tissue and viscera, the way our placenta, unraveled, would occupy miles of space. Then the image gives way to a paper fortune-teller, the intricately folded piece of paper that my friends and I played with in the cafeterias and study halls of middle school.

You fold down corner after corner, flip the paper over, and then fold corner after corner again, creating blank chambers on which to write future possibilities. You place your fingers inside and move them inward and outward, opening and closing and opening and closing, as the paper predicts what might become of you. After, you might unfold it and lay it flat on the table, but it isn't the same piece of paper. It holds something else now, imbued with hope, anxiousness, and curiosity about the future.

There is a message I am sending to my future self, my old self, a constant communication across time that lives inside my body. Pregnancy brings about the birth of not one but two new beings. Mother is not a fixed identity; we are dynamic and grow along with our young. The science of pregnancy and motherhood is just beginning to reveal the depths of our care, the extent of our own continued development.

We're unfolding, always. It's a dialogue that will last a lifetime, maybe longer, carried out within our organs, tissues, and fluids. These dispatches reverberate through the gray matter in our skulls, and maybe—if we tune in—we can hear it in our ears, feel its subtle buzz in our sinuses, as constant as the beating of our hearts.

Our bodies are the very messages that we are sending. It's about time we listen.

ACKNOWLEDGMENTS

Thank you to the scientists and caregivers so committed to improving female reproductive health for providing the foundation of this book by sharing your time, expertise, and stories with me. To Katie Hinde, in particular, for sparking a fire in my brain that I hadn't realized was there, one that I will never be able to put out. To Monika Woods, for belief and hustle. To Julie Will, for the opportunity.

For providing the space for this book to unknowingly begin, everyone at *The Stranger*, especially Kathleen Richards, whose careful editing and support made my work immeasurably better all while letting me be free, and Christopher Frizzelle, for trusting me to wander into new feature territory.

For linguistic and journalistic midwifery, solidarity, and—always—love, Jen Graves. For helping me to see early on where I was going, giving me tools to get there, and decades of stalwart friendship, Regan Kelly. For reading and believing from the very beginning, Heidi Groover and Sydney Brownstone. For free access to the many books that shaped and informed this work, the Seattle Public Library. For a back door into institutional knowledge, Heather MacLaughlin Garbes. For generosity with and at Oak Head, the most beautiful place to write, Lindy West, Ingrid West, and Ahamefule Oluo.

Many people—whether they know it or not—enabled me to write this book, including my far-flung, nebulous constellation of "Mom Friends," whose every unseen and mundane act of patience, honesty, persistence, and bravery are my inspiration: Claire Molesworth, Avi Ziv, Patty Wortham, Angie Bowlds White, Shelly Fayette, Alex Pemoulie, Jen Pham-Corbett, Danielle Thiry-Zaragoza, Rachel Kessler, Willow LeTellier, Jen Song, Amelia Abreu, Karen Neste, Bethany Miller, Erica Blake, Dawn Fornear, Danisha Christian, AyeNay Abye, Amy Garbes, Emily Zaragoza, Jill Guidi, Carly Starr, Mary Monahan, Cori Ready, Nina Mehta, Claire Tarlson, Kira Klement, Jen Magofna, Kara Hoppe, Eli Sanders, Colin Fields, Dick Dobyns, Shannon Hanks Mackey, Dalya Perez, and every person who has ever e-mailed me to tell me about their miscarriage, fears, and nipples.

For a lifetime of unwavering support, the Garbes family, especially my parents, Josie and Archimedes: Everything good in my life exists because of your love and care. Deep gratitude to the staff at El Centro de la Raza's Jose Martí Child Development Center on Beacon Hill, and Maria Oliva, as well as Gia Gillis and Fernando Ledesma, who have given my daughter safe spaces to learn and thrive, allowing me to do the same.

To Noli Jo, for making me a mom, rearranging everything, and showing me that anything is possible: It was you all along. To Ligaya Len, for teaching me even more about trust, process, and acceptance as you grew alongside this book, unconcerned for dates and deadlines, and for making our family complete.

And to Will Pittz, with more than I could ever say: For showing up at a bar one night to watch Iverson and Melo, and showing up every day since. For making this life with me, making space for this project, and never being afraid to let us become the people we are always becoming. *Sin duda*.

NOTES

INTRODUCTION

1. "Foods to Avoid During Pregnancy," WhatToExpect.com, www.whattoexpect.com/pregnancy/photo-gallery/foods-to-avoid-during-pregnancy.aspx#02.

2. William Sears and Martha Sears, *The Healthy Pregnancy Book* (New York: Little, Brown, 2013), 98–99.

3. Jordan Smith, "Oklahoma Lawmakers Want Men to Approve All Abortions," *The Intercept*, February 13, 2017, www.theintercept.com/2017/02/13/oklahoma-lawmakers-want-men-to-approve-all-abortions/.

4. Ursula K. Le Guin, "Bryn Mawr Commencement Address (1986)," *Dancing at the Edge of the World: Thoughts on Words, Women, Places* (New York: Grove Press, 1988), 160.

CHAPTER 1: NOW WHAT?

1. Randi Hutter Epstein. *Get Me Out: A History of Childbirth from the Garden of Eden to the Sperm Bank* (New York: Norton, 2010), xi.

2. Barbara Ehrenreich and Deirdre English, *For Her Own Good: Two Centuries of the Experts' Advice to Women* (New York: Anchor Books, 2005), 220.

3. ——— *Witches, Midwives, & Nurses: A History of Women Healers* (New York: The Feminist Press, 2010).

4. Ibid.

5. Tina Cassidy, *Birth: The Surprising History of How We Are Born* (New York: Grove Press, 2006).

6. Shankar Vedantam and Vanessa Northington Gamble, "Remembering Anarcha, Lucy, and Betsey: The Mothers of Modern Gynecology," National Public Radio, February 16, 2016, www.npr.org/2016/02/16/466942135/remembering-anarcha-lucy-and-betsey-the-mothers-of-modern-gynecology.

7. Ibid., xii.

8. Lynn M. Paltrow and Jeanne Flavin, "Pregnant, and No Civil Rights," *New York Times,* November 7, 2014, https://www.nytimes.com/2014/11/08/opinion/pregnant-and-no-civil-rights.html.

9. Nina Martin, "Take a Valium, Lose Your Kid, Go to Jail," *ProPublica*, September 23, 2015, www.propublica.org/article/when-the-womb-is-a-crime -scene.

10. Stephanie Clifford and Jessica Silver-Greenberg, "Foster Care as Punishment: The New Reality of 'Jane Crow,'" *New York Times*, July 21, 2017, www.nytimes .com/2017/07/21/nyregion/foster-care-nyc-jane-crow.html.

11. A. K. Summers, *Pregnant Butch: Nine Long Months Spent in Drag* (Berkeley: Soft Skull Press, 2014), 81.

12. Pew Research Center, "The American Family Today," December 14, 2015, www.pewsocialtrends.org/2015/12/17/1-the-american-family-today/.

13. Heidi Murkoff and Sharon Mazel, *What to Expect When You're Expecting*, 5th ed. (New York: Workman, 2016), 19.

CHAPTER 2: IMPERFECT CHOICES

1. Mark Sloan, *Birth Day: A Pediatrician Explores the Science, the History, and the Wonder of Childbirth* (New York: Ballantine Books, 2009), 20.

2. Ellen Gruenbaum, *The Female Circumcision Controversy: An Anthropological Perspective* (Philadelphia: University of Pennsylvania Press, 2001), 153–54. *Transactions of the Texas State Medical Association* 17 (April 1885).

3. Pliny the Elder, *Natural History*. Loeb Classical Library, doi: 10.4159/DLCL .pliny_elder-natural_history.1938, 548–49.

4. J. A. Bryant, D. G. Heathcote, and V. R. Pickles, "The Search for 'Menotoxin,'" *Lancet* 309, no. 8014 (April 1977), 753.

5. Renée Ann Cramer, *Pregnant with the Stars: Watching and Wanting the Celebrity Baby Bump* (Stanford, CA: Stanford University Press, 2015), 25.

6. Ernest L. Abel, "A Critical Evaluation of the Obstetric Use of Alcohol in Preterm Labor," *Drug and Alcohol Dependence* 7, no. 4 (July 1981).

7. Janet Lynne Golden, *Message in a Bottle: The Making of Fetal Alcohol Syndrome* (Cambridge: Harvard University Press, 2005), 55.

8. Ibid, 55.

9. Michelle Taylor, "CDC's Infographic on Women and Alcohol Goes Too Far," *Laboratory Equipment*, February 5, 2016, www.laboratoryequipment.com /blog/2016/02/cdc%E2%80%99s-infographic-women-and-alcohol-goes-too-far.

10. Ann P. Streissguth and Philippe Dehaene, "Fetal Alcohol Syndrome in Twins of Alcoholic Mothers: Concordance of Diagnosis and IQ," *American Journal of Medical Genetics* 47, no. 6 (November 1993).

11. Emily Oster, *Expecting Better: How to Fight the Pregnancy Establishment with Facts.* (New York: Penguin Press, 2013), 39.

12. Jennifer L. Payne and Samantha Meltzer-Brody, "Antidepressant Use During Pregnancy: Current Controversies and Treatment Strategies," *Clinical Obstetrics and Gynecology* 52, no. 3 (September 2009), 469–82.

13. Food and Drug Administration, "Content and Format of Labeling for Human Prescription Drug and Biological Products; Requirements for Pregnancy and Lactation Labeling," December 4, 2014, www.federalregister.gov/documents /2014/12/04/2014–28241/content-and-format-of-labeling-for-human-prescrip tion-drug-and-biological-products-requirements-for.

14. Andrew Solomon, "The Secret Sadness of Pregnancy with Depression," *New York Times Sunday Magazine*, May 28, 2015.

15. American Psychology Association, "Postpartum Depression," www.apa.org /pi/women/resources/reports/postpartum-depression.aspx.

16. Korin Miller, "Postpartum Anxiety May Be More Common Than Postpartum Depression—What You Need to Know," *Self*, April 12, 2017, www.self.com /story/postpartum-anxiety.

17. Sally Curtin and T. J. Mathews, "Smoking Prevalence and Cessation Before and During Pregnancy: Data from the Birth Certificate, 2014," *National Vital Statistics Reports* 65, no. 1 (February 10, 2016), www.cdc.gov/nchs/data/nvsr /nvsr65/nvsr65_01.pdf.

18. Marie Tae McDermott, "'It Made Me into a Person with a Mission': Readers React to Motherhood," *New York Times,* May 19, 2017, www.nytimes.com /2017/05/19/well/it-made-me-into-a-person-with-a-mission-readers-react-to -motherhood.html.

CHAPTER 3: AN ORGAN AS TWO-FACED AS TIME

1. Linda Murray, ed. *Babycenter Pregnancy: From Preconception to Birth* (New York: DK Publishing, 2010).

2. Denise Grady, "The Push to Understand the Placenta," *New York Times*, July 15, 2014.

3. D. J. Barker, "The Fetal and Infant Origins of Adult Disease," *British Medical Journal* 301, no. 6761 (November 1990), 1111.

4. J. Selander, A. Cantor, S. M. Young, and D. C. Benyshek, "Human Maternal Placentophagy: A Survey of Self-Reported Motivations and Experiences Associated with Placenta Consumption," *Ecology of Food and Nutrition* 52, no. 2 (February 2013), 93–115.

5. C. W. Coyle, K. E. Hulse, Wisner, et al., "Placentophagy: Therapeutic Miracle or Myth?" *Archives of Women's Mental Health* 18, no. 5 (October 2015), 673–80, www.ncbi.nlm.nih.gov/pmc/articles/PMC4580132/.

6. Genevieve L. Buser, Sayonara Mató, Alexia Y. Zhang, et al., "Notes from the Field: Late-Onset Infant Group B Streptococcus Infection Associated with Maternal Consumption of Capsules Containing Dehydrated Placenta—Oregon, 2016," *Morbidity and Mortality Weekly Report* 66, no. 25 (June 2017), cdc.gov /mmwr/volumes/66/wr/mm6625a4.htm?s_cid=mm6625a4_w.

7. Kathryn Schulz, "The Really Big One," *New Yorker*, July 20, 2015.

8. Robert B. Shaw, "Janus," *Poetry,* January 1971.

CHAPTER 4: BEFORE I HAD A BABY, I HAD A MISCARRIAGE

1. J. Bardos, D. Hercz, J. Friedenthal, et al., "A National Survey on Public Perceptions of Miscarriage," *Obstetrics and Gynecology* 125, no. 6 (June 2015), 1313–20.

2. Holly B. Ford and Danny J. Schust, "Recurrent Pregnancy Loss: Etiology, Diagnosis, and Therapy," *Reviews in Obstetrics and Gynecology* 2, no. 2 (Spring 2009), 76–83.

3. H. J. Janssen, M. C. Cuisinier, K. P. de Graauw, and K. A. Hoogduin, "A Prospective Study of Risk Factors Predicting Grief Intensity Following Pregnancy Loss," *Archives of General Psychiatry* 54, no. 1 (January 1997), 56–61.

CHAPTER 5: THE BEST-LAID PLANS

1. P. Douglas, "Female Sociality During the Daytime Birth of a Wild Bonobo at Luikotale, Democratic Republic of the Congo," *Primates* 55, no. 4 (October 2014): 533–42.

2. Pat Shipman, "Why Is Human Childbirth So Painful?" *American Scientist* 101, no. 6 (November–December 2013), 426.

3. American Pregnancy Association, "Calculating Conception," www.american pregnancy.org/while-pregnant/calculating-conception-due-date/.

4. Stanford Children's Health, "Calculating a Due Date," www.stanfordchil drens.org/en/topic/default?id=calculating-a-due-date-85-P01209.

5. Holly M. Dunsworth, Anna G. Warrener, Terrence Deacon, et al., "Metabolic Hypothesis for Human Altriciality," *Proceedings of the National Academy of Sciences of the United States of America* 109, no. 38 (September 2012): 15212–16.

6. Carole R. Mendelson, "Minireview: Fetal-Maternal Hormonal Signaling in Pregnancy and Labor," *Molecular Endocrinology* 23, no. 7 (July 2009): 947–54.

7. American Congress of Obstetricians and Gynecologists, "Obstetric Consensus Number One: Safe Prevention of the Primary Cesarean Delivery," March 2014, www.acog.org/Resources-And-Publications/Obstetric-Care-Consensus-Series /Safe-Prevention-of-the-Primary-Cesarean-Delivery.

8. Nina Martin and Renee Montagne, "The Last Person You'd Expect to Die in Childbirth," *ProPublica*, May 12, 2017, www.propublica.org/article/die-in-child birth-maternal-death-rate-health-care-system.

9. Ibid.

10. Centers for Disease Control and Prevention, "Advancing the Health of Mothers in the 21st Century: At a Glance 2016," www.cdc.gov/chronicdisease /resources/publications/aag/maternal.htm.

11. Allison S. Bryant, Ayaba Worjoloh, Aaron B. Caughey, and A. Eugene Washington, "Racial/Ethnic Disparities in Obstetrical Outcomes and Care: Prevalence and Determinants," *American Journal of Obstetrics Gynecology* 202, no. 4 (April 2010): 335–43, www.ncbi.nlm.nih.gov/pmc/articles/PMC2847630/pdf /nihms-169280.pdf.

12. Reynir Tómas Geirsson, "Intrauterine Volume in Pregnancy: Thesis for the Degree of Doctor Medicinae, University of Iceland 1986," *Acta Obstetricia et Gynecologica Scandinavica* 65, no. S136 (January 1986): 1–74.

13. Mark Sloan, MD, *Birth Day: A Pediatrician Explores the Science, the History, and the Wonder of Childbirth* (New York: Ballantine Books, 2009), 39–40.

14. Martin J. Blaser, *Missing Microbes* (New York: Henry Holt and Company, 2014), 93–94.

15. Josef Neu and Jona Rushing, "Cesarean versus Vaginal Delivery: Long Term Infant Outcomes and the Hygiene Hypothesis," *Clinics in Perinatology* 38, no. 2 (June 2011): 321–31, www.ncbi.nlm.nih.gov/pmc/articles/PMC3110651/.

CHAPTER 6: TAKE CARE

1. Jan Hoffman, "Estimate of U.S. Transgender Population Doubles to 1.4 Million Adults," *New York Times*, June 30, 2016, www.nytimes.com/2016/07/01/health/transgender-population.html.

2. Jessi Hempel, "My Brother's Pregnancy and the Making of a New American Family," *Time*, September 12, 2016, www.time.com/4475634/trans-man-pregnancy-evan/.

3. J. E. Soet, G. A. Brack, and C. DiIorio, "Prevalence and Predictors of Women's Experience of Psychological Trauma During Childbirth," *Birth* 30, no. 1 (March 2003): 36–46.

4. Ellen D. Hodnett, Simon Gates, G. Justus Hofmeyr, and Carol Sakala, "Continuous Support for Women During Childbirth," *Cochrane Database of Systematic Reviews* no. 7 (February 2013).

5. American Congress of Obstetricians and Gynecologists, "Obstetric Consensus Number One: Safe Prevention of the Primary Cesarean Delivery," March 2014, www.acog.org/Resources-And-Publications/Obstetric-Care-Consensus-Series/Safe-Prevention-of-the-Primary-Cesarean-Delivery.

6. Violet Beets, "The Emergence of U.S. Hospital-Based Doula Programs" (doctoral dissertation, University of South Carolina–Columbia, 2014), ProQuest Dissertations and Theses.

7. Hodnett et al., "Continuous Support for Women During Childbirth."

8. Eugene Declerq, Carol Sakala, Maureen P. Corry, et al., "Listening to Mothers III: Pregnancy and Birth, Report of the Third National U.S. Survey of Women's Childbearing Experiences," May 2013, www.transform.childbirthconnection.org/wp-content/uploads/2013/06/LTM-III_Pregnancy-and-Birth.pdf.

9. United States Department of Agriculture, "2012 Census of Agriculture Highlights: Farmers Marketing," www.agcensus.usda.gov/Publications/2012/Online_Resources/Highlights/Farmers_Marketing/Highlights_Farmers_Marketing.pdf.

10. D. A. Campbell, M. F. Lake, M. Falk, and J. R. Backstrand, "A Randomized Control Trial of Continuous Support in Labor by a Lay Doula," *Journal of Obstetric, Gynecologic & Neonatal Nursing* 35, no. 4 (July–August 2006): 456–64.

11. Louise Norris, "How Obamacare Changed Maternity Coverage," health insurance.org, August 16, 2016, www.healthinsurance.org/affordable-care-act /how-obamacare-changed-maternity-coverage/.

12. Anne Rossier Markus, Ellie Andrews, Kristina D. West, et al., "Medicaid Covered Births, 2008 Through 2010, in the Context of the Implementation of Health Reform," *Women's Health Issues* 23, no. 5 (September–October 2013): e273-80, www.whijournal.com/article/S1049–3867(13)00055–8/pdf.

13. United States Department of Labor, Bureau of Labor Statistics, "Occupational Outlook Handbook: Home Health Aides and Personal Care Aides," updated October 24, 2017, www.bls.gov/ooh/personal-care-and-service/personal -care-aides.htm.

14. Sharon Lerner, "The Real War on Families: Why the U.S. Needs Paid Leave Now," *In These Times,* August 18, 2015, inthesetimes.com/article/18151/the-real -war-on-families.

15. Bryant et al., "Racial/Ethnic Disparities in Obstetrical Outcomes and Care."

16. Rape, Abuse & Incest National Network, "Scope of the Problem: Statistics," www.rainn.org/statistics/scope-problem.

CHAPTER 7: MOTHER'S MILK

1. Susan Love, *Dr. Susan Love's Breast Book* (Boston: Da Capo Lifelong, 2015).

2. Cesar G. Victora, Rajiv Bahl, Aluisio J. D. Barros, et al., "Breastfeeding in the 21st Century: Epidemiology, Mechanisms, and Lifelong Effect," *Lancet* 387, no. 10017 (January 2016): 475–90.

3. A. Lucas, R. Morley, T. J. Cole, et al., "Breast Milk and Subsequent Intelligence Quotient in Children Born Preterm," *Lancet* 339, no. 8788 (February 1992): 261–64. Jing Yan, Lin Liu, Yun Zhu, et al., "The Association Between Breastfeeding and Childhood Obesity: A Meta-Analysis," *BMC Public Health* 14 (December 2014): 1267.

4. Olivia Ballard and Ardythe L. Morrow, "Human Milk Composition: Nutrients and Bioactive Factors," *Pediatric Clinics of North America* 60, no. 1 (February 2013): 49–74.

5. Corinne Purtill and Dan Kopf, "The Class Dynamics of Breastfeeding in the United States of America," Quartz Media LLC, July 23, 2017, qz.com/1034016 /the-class-dynamics-of-breastfeeding-in-the-united-states-of-america/.

6. Lars Bode, "Human Milk Oligosaccharides: Every Baby Needs a Sugar Mama," *Glycobiology* 22, no. 9 (September 2012): 1147–62.

7. Caroline J. Chantry, Cynthia R. Howard, and Peggy Auinger, "Full Breastfeeding Duration and Associated Decrease in Respiratory Tract Infection in US Children," *Pediatrics* 117, no. 2 (February 2006): 425–32.

8. D. T. Geddes, J. C. Kent, L. R. Mitoulas, and P. E. Hartmann, "Tongue Movement and Intra-Oral Vacuum in Breastfeeding Infants," *Early Human Development* 84, no. 7 (July 2008): 471–77.

9. Foteini Hassiotou, Anna R. Hepworth, Philipp Metzger, et al. "Maternal and Infant Infections Stimulate a Rapid Leukocyte Response in Breastmilk," *Clinical & Translational Immunology* 2, no. 4 (April 2013): e3.

10. US Department of Health and Human Services, "Diabetes Disparities Among Racial and Ethnic Minorities: Fact Sheet," (Rockville: Agency for Healthcare Research and Quality, November 2001), www.archive.ahrq.gov/research/findings /factsheets/diabetes/diabdisp/diabdisp.html.

11. K. M. Jones, M. L. Power, J. T. Queenan, et al. "Racial and Ethnic Disparities in Breastfeeding," *Breastfeeding Medicine* 10, no. 4, 186–96.

12. F. Hassiotou, A. Beltran, E. Chetwynd, et al., "Breastmilk Is a Novel Source of Stem Cells with Multilineage Differentiation Potential," *Stem Cells* 30, no. 10 (October 2012): 2164–74.

13. US Department of Health and Human Services, *Executive Summary: The Surgeon General's Call to Action to Support Breastfeeding* (Washington, DC: US Department of Health and Human Services, Office of the Surgeon General; January 20, 2011).

14. Institute of Medicine, Food and Nutrition Board, and Committee on the Evaluation of the Addition of Ingredients New to Infant Formula, *Infant Formula: Evaluating the Safety of New Ingredients* (Washington, DC: The National Academies Press, 2004).

CHAPTER 8: WHAT THIS BODY MEANS

1. Viola Polomeno, "Sex and Breastfeeding: An Educational Perspective," *Journal of Perinatal Education* 8, no. 1 (Winter 1999): 30–40.

2. Wiebke Bleidorn, Asuman Buyukcan-Tetik, Ted Schwabs, et al., "Stability and Change in Self-Esteem During the Transition to Parenthood," *Social Psychological and Personality Science* 7, no. 6 (August 2016): 560–69.

3. Kari Adamsons, "Predictors of Relationship Quality During the Transition to Parenthood," *Journal of Reproductive and Infant Psychology* 31, no. 2 (May 2013): 160–71.

4. Pew Research Center, "Parenting in America," December 17, 2015, www .pewsocialtrends.org/2015/12/17/1-the-american-family-today/.

5. "Ridgeback Slipper Lobster Molting," https://www.youtube.com/watch ?v=vqT8Dn-4L1I.

CHAPTER 9: THE SEAT OF POWER

1. Kiera Butler, "The Scary Truth About Childbirth," *Mother Jones*, January/ February 2017, www.motherjones.com/politics/2017/01/childbirth-injuries-pro lapse-cesarean-section-natural-childbirth.

2. P. G. Fernandes da Mota, A. G. Pascoal, Al Carita, and K. Bø, "Prevalence and Risk Factors of Diastasis Recti Abdominis from Late Pregnancy to 6 Months Postpartum, and Relationship with Lumbo-Pelvic Pain," *Manual Therapy* 20, no. 1 (February 2015): 200–5.

3. Butler, "The Scary Truth About Childbirth."

4. Jean M. Lawrence, E. S. Llukacz, C. W. Nager, et al., "Prevalence and Co-occurrence of Pelvic Floor Disorders in Community-Dwelling Women," *Obstetrics and Gynecology* 111, no. 3 (March 2008): 678–85.

5. D. Mazloomdoost, L. B. Westermann, C. C. Crisp, et al., "Primary Care Providers' Attitudes, Knowledge, and Practice Patterns Regarding Pelvic Floor Disorders," *International Urogynecology Journal* 28, no. 3 (March 2017): 447–53.

6. C. Glazener, A. Elders, C. Macarthur, et al., "Childbirth and Prolapse: Long-Term Associations with the Symptoms and Objective Measurement of Pelvic Organ Prolapse," *BJOG: An International Journal of Obstetrics and Gynaecology* 120, no. 2 (January 2013): 161–68.

7. H. E. O'Connell, J. M. Hutson, C. R. Anderson, and R. J. Plenter, "Anatomical Relationship Between Urethra and Clitoris," *Journal of Urology* 159, no. 6 (June 1998): 1892–97.

CHAPTER 10: UNFOLDING

1. Hilary S. Gammill, Kristina M. Adams Waldorf, Tessa M. Aydelotte, et al., "Pregnancy, Microchimerism, and the Maternal Grandmother," *PLoS ONE* 6, no. 8 (August 2011): e24101.

2. D. W. Bianchi, G. K. Zickwolf, G. J. Weil, et al. "Male Fetal Progenitor Cells Persist in Maternal Blood for as Long as 27 Years Postpartum," *Proceedings of the National Academy of Sciences of the United States of America* 93, no. 2 (January 1996): 705–8.

3. William F. N. Chan, Cécile Gumot, Thomas J. Montine, et al., "Male Microchimerism in the Human Female Brain," *PLoS ONE* 7, no. 9 (September 2012): e45592.

4. Mats Lambe, Chung-cheng Hsieh, Dimitrios Trichopoulos, et al., "Transient Increase in the Risk of Breast Cancer After Giving Birth," *New England Journal of Medicine* 331, no. 1 (July 1994): 5–9.

5. William J. Burlingham and J. Lee Nelson, "Microchimerism in Cord Blood: Mother as Anticancer Drug," *Proceedings of the National Academy of Sciences of the United States of America* 109, no. 7 (February 2012): 2190–91.

6. National Institutes of Health, "History of Congressional Appropriations, Fiscal Years 2000–2016." www.officeofbudget.od.nih.gov/pdfs/FY16/Approp%20History%20by%20IC%20FY%202000%20-%20FY%202016.pdf. Under the current administration's proposed 2018 budget, funding for all National Institutes of Health would be cut by 22 percent. "What's in Trump's 2018 Budget Request for Science?" *Science*, May 23, 2017.

7. Carl Zimmer, "A Pregnancy Souvenir: Cells That Are Not Your Own," *New York Times*, September 10, 2015.

8. American Psychology Association, "Postpartum Depression."

9. Tomas Tranströmer, "Romanesque Arches." In *The Half-Finished Heaven: The Best Poems of Tomas Tranströmer*, trans. Robert Bly (Minneapolis: Graywolf Press, 2017), 102.

ABOUT THE AUTHOR

ANGELA GARBES's writing has been featured in *New York* magazine's "The Cut" and on NPR's *Fresh Air*. She was a staff writer at the Seattle newsweekly *The Stranger*. Garbes grew up in a food-obsessed, immigrant Filipino household and now lives in Seattle with her husband and daughters.